Third Edition

Assessing Clinical Proficiencies in Athletic Training
A Modular Approach

Kenneth L. Knight, PhD, ATC, FACSM

Brigham Young University

Foreword by

Chad Starkey

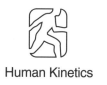

Human Kinetics

Library of Congress Cataloging-in-Publication Data

Knight, Kenneth L.
      Assessing clinical proficiencies in athletic training : a modular approach / by Kenneth
L. Knight ; foreword by Chad Starkey.-- 3rd ed.
          p. cm.
      Rev. ed. of: Clinical experiences in athletic training. 2nd ed. c1998
      Includes bibliographical references (p. 241)
      ISBN 0-7360-4199-0
      1. Physical education and training--Safety measures--Study and teaching (Higher) 2.
      Sports injuries. I. Knight, Kenneth L. Clinical experiences in athletic training. II. Title.

      GV344 .K57 2001
      617.1'027--dc21   2001039259

ISBN-10: 0-7360-4199-0
ISBN-13: 978-0-7360-4199-7

This book is a revised edition of *Clinical Experiences in Athletic Training: A Modular Approach*, published in 1998 by Human Kinetics.

Acquisitions Editor: Loarn D. Robertson, PhD; **Developmental Editor:** Myles Schrag; **Assistant Editor:** Maggie Schwarzentraub; **Copyeditor:** Julie Anderson; **Proofreader:** Sarah Wiseman; **Graphic Designer:** Robert Reuther; **Graphic Artist:** Kathleen Boudreau-Fuoss; **Cover Designer:** Stuart Cartwright; **Printer:** Edwards Brothers

Printed in the United States of America   10   9   8   7   6   5   4   3

Human Kinetics
Web site: www.HumanKinetics.com

United States: Human Kinetics
P.O. Box 5076
Champaign, IL 61825-5076
800-747-4457
e-mail: humank@hkusa.com

Canada: Human Kinetics
475 Devonshire Road Unit 100
Windsor, ON N8Y 2L5
800-465-7301 (in Canada only)
e-mail: orders@hkcanada.com

Europe: Human Kinetics
107 Bradford Road
Stanningley
Leeds LS28 6AT, United Kingdom
+44 (0) 113 255 5665
e-mail: hk@hkeurope.com

Australia: Human Kinetics
57A Price Avenue
Lower Mitcham, South Australia 5062
08 8277 1555
e-mail: liaw@hkaustralia.com

New Zealand: Human Kinetics
Division of Sports Distributors NZ Ltd.
P.O. Box 300 226 Albany
North Shore City
Auckland
0064 9 448 1207
e-mail: info@humankinetics.co.nz

Contents

Level 2: Basic Skills — 33

Level 3: Integration of Skills   117

Preface

This third edition of *Assessing Clinical Proficiencies in Athletic Training: A Modular Approach* sports a new name, is greatly expanded, and includes modules that cover all the clinical proficiencies of the 1999 National Athletic Trainers' Association (NATA) *Athletic Training Education Competencies*. Unchanged is the basic philosophy that students' clinical experiences must have structure, that learning psychomotor skills by osmosis or by just putting in time on the job is haphazard and ineffective, and that students experience too many misses under the traditional "hit-and-miss" system whereby they are required to spend 800 or 1,500 hours in the athletic training clinic developing their clinical skills.

What's New?

The new title, *Assessing Clinical Proficiencies in Athletic Training*, more fully reflects what the text has always been about: a guide to students and clinical instructors, and a pathway through the maze of psychomotor educational competencies required of entry-level athletic trainers. The purpose of this text is not to teach these skills, because there are many excellent texts that do so, but to organize these skills into a system that will help students develop the skills and will provide a measure of assessing that learning.

This edition consists of 119 modules, up from 82 in the second edition and 61 in the first edition. The new modules are the result of new educational competencies adopted by NATA in 1999 at the recommendation of the NATA Education Council.

I have rearranged the rehabilitation and advanced rehabilitation modules into therapeutic modalities and therapeutic exercise, which will more closely parallel most educational programs that teach therapeutic modalities and therapeutic exercise in separate courses.

Unfortunately for those who currently are using the program, the prefixes to most Level 2, 3, and 4 modules have changed. I apologize for the confusion that will exist during the transition into the new book. For people who are just adopting the program, the changes will make no difference. New competencies dictated additional modules and groups of modules, which could not be stacked at the end of the former ones. I hope the new and updated modules will compensate for the couple of years of slight confusion.

Also, final approval of individual modules has been adjusted in two ways. First, approved clinical instructors (ACIs) must verify completion in addition to a peer teacher. Second, grading has been removed; completing modules is an all-or-none process, and there are no B, C, or D grades.

What Is Not New?

The basic philosophy, which was innovative in 1990, has now become mainstream. The debate that raged for 15 years over how many hours athletic training students should work in order to develop sufficient skills is now over. The profession now agrees with me that developing competencies is more important than putting in hours and hoping to learn by osmosis.

The modular approach is still intact and appropriately it remains the book's subtitle. Some may choose to regroup the modules so that the program more closely fits with their curriculum. But regardless of how the modules are grouped, athletic training educators and clinical instructors can be assured that by systematically working through these modules, students will develop and demonstrate all the basic clinical skills required of entry-level athletic trainers, at least in a laboratory setting.

I also strongly support the peer teaching concept contained herein, although the program can easily be used without peer teachers if individual institutions choose to do so. But requiring students to work with younger students will reinforce the older students' knowledge and skill mastery and will decrease the "cycling" or "stuff and purge" approach to learning.

Structured Clinical Experience

For many years, athletic training educators have discussed and debated the most effective ways of teaching students the knowledge and skills necessary to be successful professionals. Much effort, time, and money have been spent in identifying the knowledge, psychomotor skills, and attitudes of professionals. As a result, we can now tell our students what knowledge, psychomotor skills, and attitudes they must master to pass the certification examination and successfully work in the field.

After many years of experience and thousands of examinations, the NATA Board of Certification has determined that athletic training skills and knowledge cannot be learned as thoroughly with on-the-job training as with a structured curriculum. Dr. Chad Starkey, a former member of the Board of Certification and presently chair of the NATA Education Council, has stated that one of the greatest needs in athletic training education is structured clinical experiences. I agree and offer a program in line with the 1999 *Athletic Training Educational Competencies* in this new edition of *Assessing Clinical Proficiencies in Athletic Training: A Modular Approach*.

Foreword

In this third edition of *Assessing Clinical Proficiencies in Athletic Training: A Modular Approach*, Kenneth L. Knight continues to build upon the qualitative approach to athletic training education that he first proposed in 1990. This advancement helps bring order to the chaos we call clinical education. The term "chaos" does not refer to the certified athletic trainer's ability to organize practice coverage, manage the facility, or even how to teach students. Chaos refers to the hit-and-miss proposition of having a student assigned to a sport or a facility in the hope that he or she will be able to acquire clinical skills based on the pathology seen. "Order" refers to providing structure to the acquisition of clinical competence that is independent from the available pathology. The student's "reward" for this effort was accruing "hours" that were applied to the eligibility to sit for the certification examination as an entry-level athletic trainer.

Athletic training clinical education is now based on the student's ability to demonstrate mastery of the clinical proficiencies. The proficiencies themselves are the integration of similar cognitive, psychomotor, and affective competencies to form a set of clinical outcomes. In other words, performing the skill only measures psychomotor competence. The proficiency measures the student's ability to integrate individual psychomotor skills into a larger objective (for example, incorporating the Lachman's test into a knee examination) and interpreting the results.

Dr. Knight's modular approach to athletic training has progressed in the past decade from a trend-setting idea to the norm in athletic training. The modular system presented in this text can be adapted to a wide range of clinical education structures. Some example structures are presented in Information for Customizing Modules (Appendix B, p. 231), but the modular nature increases its usability because it can be adapted to any clinical education structure.

The structure of Dr. Knight's text also reinforces one of the primary principles of the revised clinical education structure: learning over time. This concept represents multiple evaluations of the proficiencies in the classroom, laboratory, and clinical settings. The proficiencies are not independent from one another. Indeed, there is often overlap between one proficiency and another, assisting the learning over time process.

Our new clinical education model does not forego the traditional athletic training experiences. There is still an emphasis on practice-based education. By better preparing students in "controlled" settings, they will be better prepared to practice the art and science of athletic training in the real-world environment. By clinical instructors maximizing these experiences and capturing the "teachable moment," formal education has broken through the walls of the classroom and has spilled into athletic training rooms, clinics, and practice and game venues.

To tens of thousands of certified athletic trainers Dr. Knight forever will be remembered as the man who gave us ice. To those of us involved in athletic training pedagogy, Dr. Knight will be remembered as the man who began to bring order to the chaos that was once clinical education.

Chad Starkey, PhD, ATC
Associate Professor, Northeastern University
Chair, National Athletic Trainers' Association
Education Council

Developing Clinical Skills: Philosophy

Athletic training students must acquire practical skills. These skills require a knowledge base, but abstract knowledge is not enough—it must be applied. Skills necessary for competent sport injury management are developed only through clinical experience. The organization of the clinical experience, however, determines the depth and breadth of a student's skill development.

By Design or by Chaos

Traditionally, the underlying assumption of clinical education in athletic training, and in most other medical fields, has been that you learn by osmosis—that is, if you spend enough time "on the job," you will develop clinical skills by reacting to the situations you are exposed to.

That approach is too haphazard. Students are not all exposed to the same injuries during their clinical experiences, and therefore they do not have equal opportunities to develop clinical skills. Some sports entail many more injuries than others. And within a particular sport, the number and kinds of injuries vary from week to week and from year to year. Thus, learning from actual injuries seems to be a matter of luck.

Another problem is that student athletic trainers often waste time during team practices. Typically, there is a rush of activity immediately before practice as athletes are taped, bandaged, and cared for in preparation for the practice, and there is also much to do after practice. But unless an athlete is injured during the practice, many student athletic trainers spend practice time waiting for something to happen. If they are properly directed, student athletic trainers can use this time to develop and refine skills.

As a result, a plan was developed to ensure that all students can develop and demonstrate their competence in clinical skills that are basic to the athletic training profession, regardless of whether they are exposed to the situations requiring those skills during their clinical experiences. The result of these efforts is the modular program described in *Assessing Clinical Proficiencies in Athletic Training: A Modular Approach*. The key is to ensure that each student athletic trainer is properly directed. The modular program does this by lending structure and objectivity to the process of developing clinical skills. Athletic training educators and students can be assured that those who have properly completed the program will have had at least laboratory experience in dealing with the most common athletic injuries. Thus, the program eliminates the hit-or-miss approach to most clinical education.

Module Program Overview

The modular approach contained in this manual consists of 119 modules organized into 21 groups and four levels. Each module contains instructions to the student for developing specific skills, practicing these skills on a peer, and then demonstrating his or her competence to a peer teacher and an Approved Clinical Instructor (ACI). The individual skills or competencies were taken from the NATA 1999 *Athletic Training Education Competencies* list of clinical proficiencies required for entry-level athletic trainers.

Modules are arranged so that students begin developing simple skills and progressively acquire more complex ones. Modules are arranged into four levels and subgrouped within those levels, partly on the basis of the difficulty and complexity of the skills involved. Basic skills developed during many Level 1 and 2 modules are parts of more complex skills required for Level 3 and 4 modules.

An Integrated Curriculum

A curriculum defines a student's educational experiences. For a Council on Accreditation of Allied Health Education Programs-accredited curriculum, these are delineated by the athletic training educational competencies as well as the individual institution's philosophy and requirements (such as general education). So what is to be taught is relatively easy. But just as important is the order in which these competencies are presented to students. Students should be led through their educational experiences so that they develop foundation knowledge first and then build additional knowledge on the foundation. This program is developed to do just that.

A second concern is that skill development should be parallel to, and an outgrowth of, theory classes. In other words, skill development should be structured and integrated with presentation of theory in the classroom. Stated another way, students' clinical experiences should be a laboratory for their theory classes. Two problems arise if the two aspects are not integrated: First, students may have to develop clinical skills without adequate background or the application of theory may not be apparent. Second, students may get the idea that there are two programs, one involving the theory classes and another involving clinical experiences wherein the student develops clinical skills as an apprentice to the athletic training clinical staff.

The sequence of modules presented in this text will not parallel the theory class scheduled in all institutions. Therefore, the sequence of modules should be adjusted (as outlined in the next section) so the curriculum is integrated.

Flexibility in Program and Individual Modules

There is great variety among athletic training curriculums. Although all should teach the minimum knowledge and psychomotor skills required by the NATA education competencies, the manner in which this material is organized into a 4- or 5-year course of study is different from one institution to another. Thus, the way this modular program is adapted to individual universities will vary. Much flexibility is built into the program, which, with a little bit of foresight and planning, can be adapted to most situations.

For example, most universities want their students to learn taping and bandaging skills before modality application. Thus, taping and bandaging are grouped together here as C modules, and modality application is presented within a group of G modules. Institutions that require students to master modality application before taping may simply tell students to complete the G group of modules before the C group. One institution has redefined the levels; it has some C, some G, and some H modules together in its Level 2-1. As stated previously, skill development should be parallel to, and an outgrowth of, theory classes. So modules should parallel theory classes.

Individual institutions may elect to add additional modules or eliminate some that are contained in this manual to meet their needs and specific philosophies. Such is encouraged.

In addition to program flexibility, there also must be individual module flexibility. Most modules are totally generic, applying to students from any university. Others, such as those that deal with filling out athletic training clinic records and becoming familiar with local hospitals and physicians' offices, will be specific to each university. Procedures have been incorporated that allow specific modules to be customized to each university's situation (see p. 6 and p. 231).

Peer Teaching—Deeper Learning

Another unique aspect of this approach is that it incorporates peer teaching. Peer teachers are more advanced, more experienced students. Level 1 students look to Level 2 students as peer teachers, Level 2 students look to Level 3 students as peer teachers, and so forth. So a student can be a peer teacher (to someone less advanced) at one moment and receive peer teaching by a more advanced student the next moment.

The peer teacher's role is to help less advanced students by demonstrating, encouraging, and correcting the younger students as they practice skills. Peer teachers assist after the clinical skills, and the background information on which they are based, are taught by faculty or clinical instructors and before the student demonstrates his or her proficiency to an ACI.

Peer teaching benefits both the student who is learning as well as the peer teacher. An old adage states that the best way to learn something is to teach it. In working with younger students, peer teachers deepen their own understanding of, and ability to apply, the material. Thus, although students will demonstrate a "beginning" mastery of skills, their understanding and skills will deepen as they teach the skills to others. Such an approach helps them to learn over time; they can't just pass off a competency, forget it, and then move on to the next one.

A potential hazard of peer teaching is that if students are not conscientious when they serve as peer teachers, they may teach skills inadequately or may fail to correct a student's mistake. Over time learning may deteriorate. This can be prevented by careful supervision by clinical instructors and by a systematic and comprehensive program of oral-practical examination of all students. Such a program, outlined subsequently, helps students keep abreast of what they have learned and thus helps them be better peer teachers.

But the program can be used without peer teachers if an institution so desires. I have attempted to make the program very flexible, as described previously.

Above all, remember that peer teaching is part of mastering the skill and is not the final approval that the student has mastered the skill.

Other Advantages of This Modular Approach

In addition to ensuring that students encounter a variety of injuries and situations, this modular program provides guidelines for assigning students to specific responsibilities. With this program, students are assigned clinical duties commensurate with their skill development. Thus, students need not worry about being in over their heads, and the athletic training staff can be confident that students are able to perform assigned duties.

Using This Manual and the Modular Approach

This book contains a structured but flexible program designed to guide you through experiences that will help you develop the skills and background necessary to be a competent athletic trainer. The program will direct and assist you in practically applying the knowledge gained in didactic classes. References to the background material are part of each module, but there are many other possible sources, especially texts and journal articles from your didactic classes.

The Module Program

The program consists of 119 modules arranged into 21 blocks of related subject matter, within four levels. Each subject area is designated by a different letter:

- Modules A through M involve developing specific clinical skills.
- X modules are directed clinical experience modules.
- T modules are peer-teaching modules.
- O/P modules are oral/practical examinations.

The following section will give you an idea of the format of the modules as well as the four levels of experience, the subject matter of each block of modules, and the number of modules in each block.

Module Format

Each module consists of four parts:

- Objective or purpose of the module
- Competencies—a list of specific performance tasks or skills that you must master to reach the objective

- References—a list of one to eight texts (and page ranges within the text) that will help you refresh your knowledge of the material on which the competency is based
- Mastery and demonstration—space where your peer teacher and clinical instructor can sign when you have demonstrated to them that you are proficient in performing the competencies

Level 1: Introduction to the Clinic

1 X module: Directed Clinical Experience (Athletic Training Clinic Observation)

5 A modules: Athletic Training Clinic Operation

11 B modules: Acute Care of Injuries and Illnesses

Level 2: Basic Skills

2 X modules: Directed Clinical Experiences (Athletic Training Clinic Student Staff)

1 T module: Peer Teaching/Supervision

9 C modules: Taping, Wrapping, Bracing, and Padding

4 D modules: Risk Management

6 E modules: Basic Assessment and Evaluation

4 F modules: Basic Pharmacology and Nutrition

12 G modules: Therapeutic Modalities

16 H modules: Therapeutic Exercise

1 O/P module: O/P Examination 1

Level 3: Integration of Skills

8 X modules: Directed Clinical Experience (Team Athletic Training Staff)

2 T modules: Peer Teaching/Supervision

1 I module: Observe Surgery

18 J modules: Specific Injury Management (Prevention, Evaluation, Care, and Rehabilitation)

1 O/P module: O/P Examination 2

Level 4: Polishing Skills

2 X modules: Directed Clinical Experience (Team Student Staff)

4 T modules: Peer Teaching

3 K modules: Communication

5 L modules: Administration

3 M modules: Athletic Training Presentation

Overlap in Modules

There is some overlap in modules (for example, with anatomy in the ankle and lower leg modules). This is intentional. Modules were developed as self-contained units, so it is reasonable that some overlap would occur. Rather than look at this as extra work, look at it as an opportunity to solidify the material.

Module Completion

You can work on modules within a block (i.e., modules designated by the same letter) simultaneously and complete them in any order. In general, you must complete all modules within each block before you move to the next block of modules. Three exceptions are the F, T, and X modules: You should work on these modules at the same time you are working on other blocks within the same level.

Study, Practice, and Demonstrate Mastery

The skills included in the modules are skills you will use for a lifetime. Therefore, you should not "cycle" here (memorize, pass a test, forget the material, and move on to the next block of material). You should have been taught the material in one or more of your classes. Now is the time to solidify your knowledge and apply it. Review the material, work with peer teachers, and then practice, study, and practice. Then, when you can use the material confidently, pass it off, first to a peer teacher and then to an ACI.

Most of the time you spend working on the modules (both developing the skills and demonstrating your competence) should be during regular athletic training clinical hours; you should work with other students during "slack times." Your work on modules must not interfere with your athletic training clinical duties, but you will have a great deal of time to work on them during team meetings, practices, and so on.

Work at Your Own Pace

The program allows you to work at your own pace. However, there are a minimum and a maximum number of modules that you should complete each semester. Timing is also important, for two reasons. First, it is not fair to peer teachers to have many students come to them at the end of the semester wanting to pass off numerous modules. For most, the end of the semester is a very busy time. Second, my experience is that students sacrifice quality when they try to pass off many modules at once.

To force the issue of proper timing, Indiana State University (ISU) adopted the policy of allowing students to pass off only one module per week during the last half of the semester and none during the last week or final exams. Check with your program director concerning your program's policy.

Customizing—The Key to Flexibility

There are three ways to customize this program to individual institutional needs and preferences, and none of these ways is the "right" way. The organization of the complete curriculum, the needs of the athletic department for athletic training services, the types of equipment available, and the skills and techniques used by the full-time athletic training staff all impact the clinical education program. Most of these differences can be addressed by customizing the information in modules, adding and subtracting modules, customizing the levels and blocks of modules, and customizing the module rotation.

Customizing Modules

Most modules deal with standard or generic information and will apply to all clinical settings. Others, however, involve specifics that vary from one university to another and therefore will need to be customized. For instance, Module A2 pertains to record keeping; because most universities use their own forms, you need to become familiar with the forms and record-keeping system of your program.

The following modules require customizing:

• **A2 Injury Record Keeping:** Records and forms used in your athletic training clinics, such as daily treatment logs, individual treatment sheets, insurance forms, and referral to physician

• **A3 Athletic Training Supplies:** Selected medical supplies used during this module to acquaint you with the types of supplies used in the athletic training clinic and with how they are inventoried, purchased, stored, and made accessible for daily use

• **A4 Athletic Training Clinic Equipment—Small:** Selected medical equipment used during this module to acquaint you with the types of small equipment (braces, pads, etc.) used in the athletic training clinic and with how the items are inventoried, purchased, stored, and made accessible for daily use

• **A5 Athletic Training Clinic Equipment—Major:** Major equipment (such as ice machines and therapeutic modalities) used during this module to familiarize you with the types of major equipment used in the athletic training clinic and with how it is purchased

• **B5 Medical Services (Health Centers, Hospitals, Physicians):** Names of community medical services to which athletic training students may need to transport athletes, such as physicians' offices, hospital emergency rooms, and hospital outpatient surgical units

• **H6 Isotonic Strength-Training Devices:** Weight-training equipment that athletic training students use in athletic training clinics for rehabilitation, including at least one piece of equipment for each major joint of the body

Modules to Ignore or Add

Some modules in this book may not apply to your athletic training program, and there may be additional modules that your curriculum director or head athletic trainer has written specifically for you. Obtain these from your curriculum director or head athletic trainer.

Customizing Module Levels and Blocks

Institutional philosophy and how your theory classes are organized and taught will dictate differences in the order that you develop clinical skills. The order and grouping of modules may be customized to fit individual institutional philosophy.

Customizing Module Rotation

Universities with clinical education phases ranging from 2+ to 4 years have adopted this program. The table shows possible schedules for work on the five levels within clinical education sequences of different lengths; I'm sure there are other possibilities.

How Do You Know What Is Customized?

Your athletic training curriculum director or head athletic trainer will supply you with the appropriate information for the modules listed. He or she may use one or more of the lists supplied in appendix B or may have information sheets specific to your situation. Get the needed information from him or her.

Possible Schedules for Progression Through the Four Clinical Proficiency Levels for Various Program Lengths				
	LEVEL			
Program length	**1**	**2**	**3**	**4**
2½ years	1st semester	2nd and 3rd semesters	3rd and 4th semesters	5th semester
3 years	1st semester	2nd and 3rd semesters	4th and 5th semesters	6th semester
3½ years	1st semester	2nd and 3rd semester	4th and 5th semesters	6th and 7th semesters
4 years	1st semester	2nd, 3rd, and 4th semesters	4th, 5th, and 6th semesters	7th and 8th semesters

When Do You Work on Modules?

You may demonstrate your mastery of module competencies during regular athletic training clinic work hours. You should make arrangements ahead of time with an appropriate module supervisor. Allow extra time in case an emergency arises that would require your or your supervisor's services in caring for athletes. Before your conference with a module supervisor, check the references at the end of this book, practice the individual skills of the module, practice testing, and then practice demonstrating all module skills to a peer.

Module supervisors include athletic training faculty and students at your college or university. Students may supervise and sign for module work at a level they have completed. For example, a person at Level 3 can supervise people working on Levels 1 and 2.

Customized Reference Library

Each module includes selected references. The full citations for these references are provided at the end of this text. But there are many other excellent references for this material. Your athletic training program should maintain a library of these additional references. Find out where they are kept. As you complete your education, add to the list as you find great references. The following are examples of additional references used by Oregon State University for its module on bloodborne pathogens:

- The 1995 NATA *Position Statement on Bloodborne Pathogens*
- Oregon Occupational Health and Safety Administration (OSHA) Bloodborne Pathogens Regulations
- The American Liver Foundation lay summaries on hepatitis A, B, and C
- The June 1996 Oregon State University Safety Bulletin *Tuberculosis and Infection Control in the Workplace*

Oral/Practical Examinations

Oral/practical (O/P) examinations are an excellent way of assisting and motivating students to develop clinical skills. Broad comprehensive O/P examina-

tions should be given at key points in the program to assess students' retention of the skills they have learned up to that point in the program. In addition, mini O/P exams every 3 to 4 weeks help students keep up to date on material they have mastered. Thus, O/P exams are an additional way of helping students learn over time. Obviously, students don't have to review the skills they use more often in the clinic, but those skills that they do not use regularly will be lost without periodic review and repetition.

There are other benefits to incorporating O/P exams in the curriculum. First, they help student with their peer teaching. By keeping current with their newly developed skills, students have a stronger knowledge base from which to teach. A second benefit from periodic O/P exams is that they help students perform under pressure, which often is a part of real-life situations when athletes are injured during crucial athletic contests. A third benefit is that O/P exams help prepare students psychologically for the NATA Board of Certification (NATABOC) examination.

I have found success in organizing mini O/P exams as follows. Mini exams are given every 3 weeks during the weekly "practicum class." Students are divided into groups of five, all within the same level. Each group is given three copies of five different O/P questions. The students draw lots to determine their order: Number 1 is the examinee, 2 is the model, and 3, 4, and 5 are the examiners. The examiners then administer the first exam. After the first exam is completed, the students shift positions and the second exam is given, and so on until all five group members have been examined. In less than an hour, all students can be tested, each at his or her own level. Clinical instructors rotate from group to group to monitor the exams.

Two comprehensive O/P exams are built into this program—one after Level 2 and another after Level 3. More could be given, but I discourage less than two. These can be administered by faculty or peers; I have done both for more than 20 years and find benefits to both methods. I organize O/P exams on a single day, with each student scheduled for a 30- to 40-minute exam, and multiple exams occurring in different rooms. When I use peer examiners, I always have faculty or ACIs administer the first few exams, and students rotate into being an examiner after they have been tested themselves. Typically they are involved in five exams: one as the examinee, one as the model, and three as an examiner. When the exams are administered by peers, I always have an ACI closely monitor the examination sites. The important thing is that the exams are comprehensive and students know they must prepare for such.

Students find that giving exams is also an important learning experience. They frequently recognize aspects of the skill they may have forgotten. And students see firsthand the effects of pressure on performance and the need for constant repetition, when peers forget critical aspects of a skill that they were able to perform in a group study session the previous night.

Appendix C contains the instructions and some of the questions developed during 18 years of giving O/P examinations at ISU.

Level 1

Introduction
to the Clinic

The first groups of modules are designed to help athletic training students begin their clinical education. Working on these modules will help them understand what an athletic training clinic is, how it operates, and how it interfaces with the larger world of athletic health care. Students also will demonstrate proficiency in basic emergency and acute care of athletic injuries.

Note: The term *clinic* as used herein refers to any facility where athletic health care is administered. Clinic is defined as "a center for physical examination and treatment of ambulant patients who are not hospitalized (*Tabers Cyclopedic Dictionary*, 16th ed.). Most athletic departments call the place that athletic trainers perform their labors a "training room," even though it often is a suite of rooms, and there is little "training" going on there. I believe that *athletic injury clinic, sports medicine clinic*, or *athletic health clinic* more appropriately describe what goes on there. It is an allied healthcare facility and should be referred to as such. I will use the term *athletic training clinic* here, which has elements of the past yet recognizes that the facility is a health facility.

Level 1 includes 17 modules, organized into three groups:

Athletic Training Observation

Objective

Become familiar with the clinical aspect of the athletic training profession.

Competencies

1. Spend at least 50 hours observing the activities and operation of an athletic training clinic. You will be assigned specific times that you are to attend, and you may be assigned to different athletic training clinics if your college has more than one. Keep track of your time on a time sheet provided by your program director.

2. Interview at least two staff athletic trainers and write a brief report of that interview. Include in your report things such as what a typical day is like, the worst day they have had, the kind of day they hope they will never have, their best day, why they chose athletic training as a career, what they like most and dislike most about their careers, what they might do differently if they could start over, and so forth.

3. Write, in the form of a journal manuscript, a case report of an injured athlete whom you observe during these experiences. See the "Authors Guide" of the *Journal of Athletic Training* for specific guidelines and tips. You can find this guide in any issue of the *Journal of Athletic Training* or from the journal Web site: **www.journalofathletictraining.com**. Your report should cover at least 3 weeks and contain the pertinent events and information concerning an athlete's injury, the care provided, and how this case relates to suggested protocols given in standard athletic training texts. In each report include the following:

   a. A brief introduction in which you state why you selected the case

   b. Personal data (age, sex, race, marital status, and occupation when relevant, but not name)

   c. Chief complaint and history of present complaint (including symptoms)

   d. Results of physical examination (e.g., "Physical findings relevant to the rehabilitation program were…")

   e. Medical history (surgery, laboratory results, exam, and so on)

   f. Diagnosis

   g. Treatment and clinical course (immediate care and rehabilitation, including specific dates or times)

   h. Criteria for return to competition

   i. How the athlete handled competition

   j. A discussion in which you compare and contrast this case with protocols published in standard athletic training texts

References

Your athletic training department's staff athletic trainers

The *Journal of Athletic Training*, published quarterly by NATA. See NATA's Web site at **www.nata.com**.

Texts listed in the reference section of this manual, p. 241.

Mastery and Demonstration

Master these competencies by reviewing your class notes and texts, observing peer teachers and certified/licensed professionals perform the skills, discussing the competencies with peer teachers and certified/licensed professionals, practicing alone and with a peer, and then demonstrating proficiency to a peer teacher. Finally, demonstrate your proficiency to an ACI.

Module X1—Athletic Training Observation (continued)

Approved by (date and signature)   **Comments**

  1. Time sheet

      Peer _____

      ACI _____

  2. Interview

      Peer _____

      ACI _____

  3. Case Report

      Peer _____

      ACI _____

Athletic Training Clinic Operations

Administrative Policies and Procedures

Objective

Become familiar with the responsibilities, policies, and procedures of your college/university athletic training department.

Competencies

1. Identify and discuss each athletic training and sports medicine facility at your university. In your discussion, include the following:

   a. Name and location of the facility

   b. Primary purpose or goal of the facility

   c. The typical daily schedule of activities at the facility

   d. The staff, graduate assistants, and student athletic trainers assigned to the facility

2. Describe the regular (daily and weekly) cleaning and maintenance responsibilities of student and staff athletic trainers at each facility.

3. Read your athletic training department's administrative policies and procedures manual. Then discuss its major points with a peer teacher.

References

Your athletic training department

Mastery and Demonstration

Practice and reinforce these competencies by reviewing your class notes and texts, observing peer teachers and certified/licensed professionals perform the skills, discussing the competencies with peer teachers and certified/licensed professionals, practicing alone and with a peer, and then demonstrating proficiency to a peer teacher. Finally, demonstrate your proficiency to an ACI.

Approved by (date and signature)

1. Facilities

   Peer _____ Michael Slater _____

   ACI _____

2. Maintenance

   Peer _____ M S _____

   ACI _____

3. Policies and procedures manual

   Peer _____ M S _____

   ACI _____

Comments

Injury Record Keeping

Objective

Learn why record keeping is essential to athletic training clinic operations and how to keep such records; demonstrate the ability to maintain records with sensitivity to patient confidentiality.

Competencies

1. Discuss how proper record keeping is important in the following areas:

   a. Improving athletes' health care

   b. Communicating among staff

   c. Communicating with insurance companies

   d. Preventing lawsuits

2. Discuss why patient confidentiality is a necessary part of injury record keeping, and discuss three ways of ensuring patient confidentiality.

3. Demonstrate your ability to select and use standardized record-keeping methods by comparing and contrasting the major aspects of the SOAP, HIPS, and HOPS systems of injury record keeping.

4. For each of the records listed subsequently (a-f), do the following:

   • Discuss the purpose of the record

   • Demonstrate how to properly fill it out

   • Discuss where and how long the record is filed short term   7yrs

   • Discuss where and how long the record is filed long term

   a. Injury

   b. Rehabilitation

   c. Physician referral

   d. Insurance documentation

   e. Individual progress notes

   f. Coach's updates

5. Demonstrate your ability to organize patient files to allow systematic storage and retrieval.

6. Demonstrate your ability to properly enter data into your athletic training clinic's injury software program. (If your clinic does not use injury software, obtain a brochure for a contemporary program and describe its major features.)

References

Your athletic training department

Arnheim and Prentice 2000 (pp. 52-60)

Rankin and Ingersoll 2001 (pp. 124-180)

Ray 2000 (pp. 159-191)

Mastery and Demonstration

Practice and reinforce these competencies by reviewing your class notes and texts, observing peer teachers and certified/licensed professionals perform the skills, discussing the competencies with peer teachers and certified/licensed professionals, practicing alone and with a peer, and then demonstrating proficiency to a peer teacher. Finally, demonstrate your proficiency to an ACI.

Approved by (date and signature)

1. Importance

   Peer _Anastasia J White_ 12/7

   ACI _____

2. Confidentiality

   Peer _AJW_ _____

   ACI _____

3. Standardized

   Peer _AJW_ _____

   ACI _____

Module A2—Injury Record Keeping (continued)

4a. Injury

　　 Peer _____

　　 ACI _____

4b. Rehabilitation

　　 Peer _____

　　 ACI _____

4c. Physician referral

　　 Peer _____

　　 ACI _____

4d. Insurance documentation

　　 Peer _____

　　 ACI _____

4e. Individual progress notes

　　 Peer _____

　　 ACI _____

4f. Coach's updates

　　 Peer _____

　　 ACI _____

5. Record storage

　　 Peer _____

　　 ACI _____

6. Computer software

　　 Peer _____

　　 ACI _____

Comments

Athletic Training Supplies

Objectives

Become familiar with the purpose/function of medical supplies commonly used by athletic trainers and how these supplies are purchased, inventoried, stored, and used at your university.

Competencies

1. Discuss the purpose/use of the athletic training/medical supplies on the list supplied by your clinical supervisor. (Note: This short list of items is intended as a random sampling of your knowledge and understanding of where athletic training supplies and equipment are kept, as well as their intended function. The list is not all-inclusive!)

2. Locate one of each item from the list in Competency 1 in the daily work area of your athletic training clinic and from the bulk storage area.

3. Discuss your university's plan for restocking supplies in work areas (shelves and treatment/taping areas) with the supplies used there.

4. Assist others in restocking supplies on three separate days.

5. Browse through at least two athletic training/medical supply catalogs. As you do so, identify five items in each catalog that are in your supply room/area and three items that are not used at your university.

6. Explain the annual inventory process used by your athletic training department. Explain how each form is filled out.

References

Catalogs on file in your athletic training clinic office or library

Mastery and Demonstration

Practice and reinforce these competencies by reviewing your class notes and texts, observing peer teachers and certified/licensed professionals perform the skills, discussing the competencies with peer teachers and certified/licensed professionals, practicing alone and with a peer, and then demonstrating proficiency to a peer teacher. Finally, demonstrate your proficiency to an ACI.

Approved by (date and signature)

1. Supply use
   Peer _Bethany Hyde_____
   ACI _____

2. Supply stores
   Peer _BH_____
   ACI _____

3. Restock plan
   Peer _BH_____
   ACI _____

4. Restock
   Peer _BH_____
   ACI _____

5. Catalogs
   Peer _BH_____
   ACI _____

6. Inventory
   Peer _BH_____
   ACI _____

Comments

Athletic Training Clinic Equipment—Small

Objective

Become familiar with the purpose/function of medical equipment commonly used by athletic trainers and how these supplies are purchased, inventoried, stored, and used at your university.

Competencies

1. Discuss the purpose/use of the athletic training/medical equipment on the list supplied by your clinical supervisor. (Note: This short list of items is intended as a random sampling of your knowledge and understanding of where athletic training supplies and equipment are kept, as well as their intended function. The list is not all-inclusive!)

2. Locate one of each item from the list in Competency 1 in the daily work area of your athletic training clinic and/or from the bulk storage area.

3. Discuss your university's plan for distributing these equipment items to athletes. Which items are considered disposable, and which are returned by the athlete for reuse by someone else?

4. Browse through at least two athletic training/medical supply catalogs. As you do so, identify five items in each catalog that are in your supply room/area and three items that are not used at your university.

References

Catalogs on file in your athletic training clinic office or library

Mastery and Demonstration

Practice and reinforce these competencies by reviewing your class notes and texts, observing peer teachers and certified/licensed professionals perform the skills, discussing the competencies with peer teachers and certified/licensed professionals, practicing alone and with a peer, and then demonstrating proficiency to a peer teacher. Finally, demonstrate your proficiency to an ACI.

Approved by (date and signature)

1. Purpose

   Peer _____

   ACI _____

2. Storage

   Peer _____

   ACI _____

3. Distribution

   Peer _____

   ACI _____

4. Purchase

   Peer _____

   ACI _____

Comments

Athletic Training Clinic Equipment—Major

Objective

To become familiar with the names, locations, and uses of the medical instruments/machines used to treat and rehabilitate injured athletes.

Competencies

1. As you stroll through your athletic training clinic, name each piece of medical equipment and explain its major purpose.

2. Browse through at least two athletic training/medical equipment catalogs. As you do so, identify two types of equipment in each catalog that are used in your athletic training clinic and two types that are not used at your university.

References

Catalogs on filex in your athletic training clinic office or library

Mastery and Demonstration

Practice and reinforce these competencies by reviewing your class notes and texts, observing peer teachers and certified/licensed professionals perform the skills, discussing the competencies with peer teachers and certified/licensed professionals, practicing alone and with a peer, and then demonstrating proficiency to a peer teacher. Finally, demonstrate your proficiency to an ACI.

Approved by (date and signature)

1. Purpose

   Peer _____

   ACI _____

2. Purchase

   Peer _____

   ACI _____

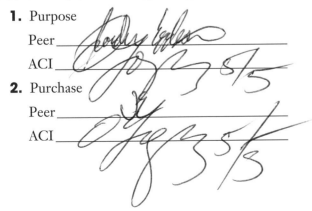

Comments

Acute Care of Injuries and Illnesses

Implement Emergency Action Plan

Objective

Demonstrate ability to implement an emergency action plan (EAP) for an activity, setting, or event.

Competencies

1. Obtain a copy of the EAPs from your athletic training department's policies and procedures manual. Discuss in detail the key elements of one of these EAPs.

2. Explain "triage" and explain how you would triage in an emergency situation with numerous injuries of various seriousness.

References

Hillman 2000 (pp. 280-301)

Pfeiffer and Mangus 1998 (pp. 75-81)

Mastery and Demonstration

Practice and reinforce these competencies by reviewing your class notes and texts, observing peer teachers and certified/licensed professionals perform the skills, discussing the competencies with peer teachers and certified/licensed professionals, practicing alone and with a peer, and then demonstrating proficiency to a peer teacher. Finally, demonstrate your proficiency to an ACI.

Approved by (date and signature)

1. EAP

Peer _____

ACI _____

2. Triage

Peer _____

ACI _____

Comments

Acute Care of Injuries and Illnesses

Cardiopulmonary Resuscitation

Objective

To be able to perform rescue breathing and external chest compressions if necessary to prolong life.

Competencies

1. Demonstrate your competence in cardiopulmonary resuscitation (CPR) by having a valid American Red Cross or American Heart Association CPR card.

2. If the following tasks were not part of your CPR training, demonstrate them:

   a. Establish and manage an airway in an athlete wearing protective headgear.

   b. Perform CPR on an adult or child with or without a spinal injury.

   c. Use a bag-valve-mask on an adult or child for rescue breathing.

   d. Use a protective pocket mask/shield on an adult or child for rescue breathing.

   e. Demonstrate two-person CPR to assist a drowning victim.

3. Discuss how long your CPR certification is valid, how you can become recertified, and the NATA continuing education requirement for CPR.

References

American Red Cross or American Heart Association

Hillman 2000 (pp. 271-274, 297-301)

Pfeiffer and Mangus 1998 (pp. 267-282)

Mastery and Demonstration

Practice and reinforce these competencies by reviewing your class notes and texts, observing peer teachers and certified/licensed professionals perform the skills, discussing the competencies with peer teachers and certified/licensed professionals, practicing alone and with a peer, and then demonstrating proficiency to a peer teacher. Finally, demonstrate your proficiency to an ACI.

Approved by (date and signature)

1. CPR certified

   Peer _____Michall Slate_____

   ACI _____

2a. Airway/headgear

   Peer _____MS_____

   ACI _____

2c. Bag-valve-mask

   Peer _____MS_____

   ACI _____

2d. Pocket mask/shield

   Peer _____MS_____

   ACI _____

2e. Two-person CPR

   Peer _____MS_____

   ACI _____

Comments

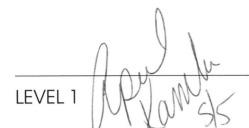

Module B3

Acute Care of Injuries and Illnesses

Choking, Hemorrhaging, and Shock

Objective

Develop and demonstrate the skills necessary to properly recognize and manage choking, severe hemorrhage, and shock.

Competencies

1. Discuss choking, when you would use each of the following, and demonstrate the following:

   a. Heimlich maneuver, standing

   b. Heimlich maneuver, lying

   c. Finger sweep

2. Discuss why severe hemorrhaging is a medical emergency, how to control it, and demonstrate the following:

   a. Tourniquet application

   b. Direct pressure

3. Discuss shock, how you would treat a patient in shock, and the consequences of not properly treating such a patient.

Loss of Fluids

References

Arnheim and Prentice 2000 (pp. 282-286)

Pfeiffer and Mangus 1998 (pp. 80-81, 274-277)

A first aid book

Mastery and Demonstration

Practice and reinforce these competencies by reviewing your class notes and texts, observing peer teachers and certified/licensed professionals perform the skills, discussing the competencies with peer teachers and certified/licensed professionals, practicing alone and with a peer, and then demonstrating proficiency to a peer teacher. Finally, demonstrate your proficiency to an ACI.

Approved by (date and signature)

1. Choking

   Peer _Michael Staley_

   ACI _____

2. Hemorrhaging

   Peer _____ M S _____

   ACI _____

3. Shock

   Peer _____ M S _____

   ACI _____

Comments

Shock- Imblane of homeostais

lowe bp
over breathing
rapid but weak pulse
Blue skin

Change in metal status

Emergency Transportation

Objective

To be able to transport athletes from the field or court after injuries of various degrees of seriousness.

Competencies

1. Explain the procedures for obtaining an ambulance for the following:

a. An athlete at your university

b. A nonathlete university student

2. Demonstrate proper care of an athlete with a suspected spinal injury including stabilization and spine board or body splint.

3. Demonstrate proper transportation off the field without a stretcher (e.g., manual conveyance technique for a sprained ankle or knee).

4. Demonstrate proper selection and application of splints (traditional, air, or vacuum) for the following:

a. Dislocated talus

b. Fractured midhumerus

c. Fractured distal radius

d. Fractured distal tibia

e. Subluxated patella

f. Sprained elbow

References

AAOS 1999 (pp. 221, 703)

Anderson, Hall, and Martin 2000 (pp. 90-92)

Arnheim and Prentice 2000 (pp. 293-302)

Hillman 2000 (pp. 275-301)

Pfeiffer and Mangus 1998 (pp. 63, 109-118)

Starkey and Ryan 2002 (pp. 647-650)

Mastery and Demonstration

Practice and reinforce these competencies by reviewing your class notes and texts, observing peer teachers and certified/licensed professionals perform the skills, discussing the competencies with peer teachers and certified/licensed professionals, practicing alone and with a peer, and then demonstrating proficiency to a peer teacher. Finally, demonstrate your proficiency to an ACI.

Approved by (date and signature)

1. Ambulance

Peer_____

ACI_____

2. Spinal injury

Peer_____

ACI_____

3. Transportation without stretcher

Peer_____

ACI_____

4. Splints

Peer_____

ACI_____

Comments

Acute Care of Injuries and Illnesses

Medical Services
(Health Center, Hospitals, Physicians)

Objective

To become familiar with the facilities and personnel of the various medical facilities that you will encounter while caring for injured athletes.

Competencies

Complete a tour of your university student health center, hospital, or clinic where athletes are cared for when they need care beyond what you can administer in the athletic training clinic. Have the person conducting the tour sign in the following space. In addition, write the name and phone number of each of the following health center personnel. (Note: See if any of these positions have different titles at your university. If so, write the correct title in place of the incorrect one in the following list.)

Tour Director _____

    Ph_____

Health Center Director _____

    Ph_____

Assistant Director _____

    Ph_____

Physician _____

    Ph_____

Physician _____

    Ph_____

Physician _____

    Ph_____

Physician _____

    Ph_____

Head Nurse _____

    Ph_____

Assistant Head Nurse _____

    Ph_____

Pharmacist _____

    Ph_____

X-ray Technician _____

    Ph_____

References

A peer teacher

Mastery and Demonstration

Complete a tour of the previously mentioned facilities and discuss the highlights of each tour with a peer teacher and then an ACI.

Tour Date _____

Peer _____

ACI _____

Comments

Acute Care of Injuries and Illnesses

Rest, Ice, Compression, Elevation, and Support

Objective

Compression- like a tight sock.

Develop and demonstrate the skills necessary to provide appropriate initial care for acute sprains, strains, and contusions.

every hours

Competencies

1. Demonstrate application of rest, ice, compression, elevation, and support (RICES) for initial care of the following conditions. Indicate how long each should be applied and reapplied and criteria for removal.

   a. Sprained ankle

   b. Strained hamstring

   c. Dislocated finger

   d. Dislocated shoulder (four separate injuries)

2. Demonstrate your ability to help an athlete use crutches by properly fitting the crutches, instructing the athlete in proper crutch walking technique (both swing and three-point gaits), coaching the athlete as he or she practices walking, and correcting the athlete as necessary. Tell when to use each gait and how to help an athlete progress to normal walking.

3. Demonstrate application of two different types of slings (one using elastic wraps) to an athlete with a shoulder injury.

   a. Elastic wrap sling

   b. Nonelastic wrap sling

References

Arnheim and Prentice 2000 (pp. 290-291, 302-303)

Knight 1995 (pp. 85-98, 209-215)

Mastery and Demonstration

Practice and reinforce these competencies by reviewing your class notes and texts, observing peer teachers and certified/licensed professionals perform the skills, discussing the competencies with peer teachers and certified/licensed professionals, practicing alone and with a peer, and then demonstrating proficiency to a peer teacher. Finally, demonstrate your proficiency to an ACI.

Approved by (date and signature)

1a. RICES—sprained ankle

Peer _____

ACI _____

1b. RICES—strained hamstring

Peer _____

ACI _____

1c. RICES—dislocated finger

Peer _____

ACI _____

1d. RICES—dislocated shoulder

Peer _____

ACI _____

2. Crutch use

Peer _____

ACI _____

3a. Sling—elastic wrap

Peer _____

ACI _____

3b. Sling—nonelastic wrap

Peer _____

ACI _____

Comments

Open Wounds

Objective

Develop and demonstrate the skills necessary to provide appropriate initial care to open wounds.

Competencies

1. Define and explain how each of the following types of open wounds occurs during athletic activities:

   a. Abrasion

   b. Laceration

   c. Puncture

   d. Incision

   e. Avulsion

2. For each of the types of wounds in Competency 1, demonstrate and explain the following:

   - Use universal precautions
   - Stop bleeding with direct and indirect pressure
   - Cleanse the wound
   - Disinfect the wound
   - Treat the wound with ointment
   - Dress the wound
   - Protect the wound during practice/competition
   - Manage the wound through healing

3. For each of the types of wounds in Competency 1, tell what signs or symptoms would be cause for concern. How would you deal with each of the concerns?

Call 911 with indirect pressure

References

Anderson, Hall, and Martin 2000 (pp. 108-112)

Arnheim and Prentice 2000 (pp. 739-751)

Foster, Rowedder, and Reese 1995

Hillman 2000 (pp. 297-306)

Knight 1995 (pp. 247-249)

Pfeiffer and Mangus 1998 (pp. 229-231)

Rheinecker 1995

Mastery and Demonstration

Practice and reinforce these competencies by reviewing your class notes and texts, observing peer teachers and certified/licensed professionals perform the skills, discussing the competencies with peer teachers and certified/licensed professionals, practicing alone and with a peer, and then demonstrating proficiency to a peer teacher. Finally, demonstrate your proficiency to an ACI.

Approved by (date and signature)

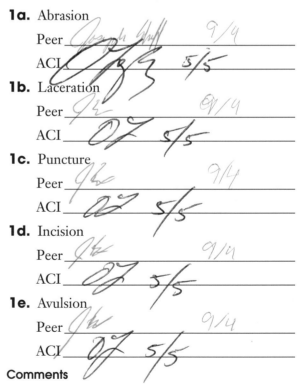

1a. Abrasion

Peer _____ 9/4

ACI _____ 5/5

1b. Laceration

Peer _____ 9/4

ACI _____ 5/5

1c. Puncture

Peer _____ 9/4

ACI _____ 5/5

1d. Incision

Peer _____ 9/4

ACI _____ 5/5

1e. Avulsion

Peer _____ 9/4

ACI _____ 5/5

Comments

Due Sept 30

10:1 bleach
viralcide
fungalcide

Acute Care of Injuries and Illnesses

Universal Precautions Against Bloodborne Pathogens, Hepatitis, and Tuberculosis

Objective

Understand and be able to apply the federal OSHA bloodborne pathogens standards (laws).

Competencies → *written assign*

1. Define the following terms:
   a. Bloodborne pathogens
   b. Contaminated laundry
   c. Contaminated sharps
   d. Exposure incident
   e. Exposure control plan
   f. Handwashing facilities
   g. Occupational exposure
   h. Other potentially infectious materials
   i. Personal protective equipment
   j. Source individual
   k. Universal precautions
   l. Hepatitis A
   m. Hepatitis B
   n. Hepatitis C
   o. Tuberculosis

2. Locate where the sharps containers, supply of rubber gloves, and chlorine bleach or other acceptable disinfectants are kept in each athletic training clinic you will work in during your student athletic training career. Discuss the benefits and limitations of these methods of protection.

3. Demonstrate how you would mix an effective solution to disinfect a wrestling mat or examination table of potential human immunodeficiency virus (HIV) contamination after an athlete has bled on it. What would you do with the materials (towels, sponges, and the like) you used to clean the mat?

4. Explain the methods of transmission of HIV and hepatitis B that place allied healthcare workers at risk. Describe the methods of transmission of hepatitis A and hepatitis C and the types of precautions you would take in your role as a student athletic trainer to protect yourself from transmission.

5. Using a student volunteer and all the appropriate supplies and equipment, simulate how you would debride an open (bleeding) wound in an athlete, given what you now know about the OSHA guidelines and HIV/hepatitis transmission.

6. Define tuberculosis (TB) and describe how the disease is spread. Describe the four types of control measures to be taken by workers who are at risk for occupational exposure to TB.

References

AAOS 1999 (pp. 632-652)

American Liver Foundation summaries on hepatitis A, B, and C

Arnheim and Prentice 2000 (pp. 322-342)

Arnold 1995

NATA Position Statement: Bloodborne Pathogens

Pfeiffer and Mangus 1998 (pp. 283-312)

Rheinecker 1995

Starkey and Ryan 2002 (pp.22-26)

Mastery and Demonstration

Practice and reinforce these competencies by reviewing your class notes and texts, observing peer teachers and certified/licensed professionals perform the skills, discussing the competencies with

Module B8—Universal Precautions Against Bloodborne Pathogens, Hepatitis, and Tuberculosis (continued)

peer teachers and certified/licensed professionals, practicing alone and with a peer, and then demonstrating proficiency to a peer teacher. Finally, demonstrate your proficiency to an ACI.

Comments

Approved by (date and signature)

1. Term definitions

Peer _Bethany Hyde_____

ACI _____

2. Equipment location

Peer _BH_____

ACI _____

3. Disinfectant solution

Peer _BH_____

ACI _____

4. Disease transmission

Peer _BH_____

ACI _____

5. Wound debridement

Peer _BH_____

ACI _____

6. TB and control

Peer _BH_____

ACI _____

Acute Care of Injuries and Illnesses

Environmental Injury/Illness

Objective

Develop and demonstrate the skills necessary to properly recognize and manage selected environment-related injuries and illnesses.

Competencies

1. Discuss the conditions and situations related to the following environmental factors that are potentially hazardous to athletes. Discuss appropriate recommendations for sports activity to lessen the potential for injury.
    a. Heat — cramps, exashion, stroke
    b. Humidity
    c. Cold
    d. Wind
    e. Lightning strike
    f. Poor air quality

2. Demonstrate and explain the proper use of the following and how to interpret data from these items:
    a. A sling psychrometer
    b. A wet bulb globe index

3. Explain the signs, symptoms, and proper management of the following:
    a. Heat cramps
    b. Heat exhaustion
    c. Heat syncope — pass out
    d. Heat stroke
    e. Hypothermia

4. Explain physical and environmental factors that are potential hazards for athletes partici-

pating in the following activity settings. Also, tell how and how often you should check each.
    a. Basketball court
    b. Football field
    c. Soccer field
    d. Softball field
    e. Volleyball court

5. Explain how to use and interpret weight charts. For which sports are weight charts most important? See weight diff from water loss

References

AAOS 1999 (pp. 654-663)

Anderson, Hall, and Martin 2000 (pp. 532-549)

Arnheim and Prentice 2000 (pp. 139-158)

Hillman 2000 (pp. 205-231)

NATA Position Statement: Lightning Safety

NATA Position Statement: Fluid Replacement for Athletes

Pfeiffer and Mangus 1998 (pp. 242-251)

Starkey and Ryan 2002 (pp. 653-666)

Mastery and Demonstration

Practice and reinforce these competencies by reviewing your class notes and texts, observing peer teachers and certified/licensed professionals perform the skills, discussing the competencies with peer teachers and certified/licensed professionals, practicing alone and with a peer, and then demonstrating proficiency to a peer teacher. Finally, demonstrate your proficiency to an ACI.

Module B9—Environmental Injury/Illness (continued)

Approved by (date and signature)   **Comments**

1. Environmental hazards

Peer _____

ACI _____

2. Devices

Peer _____

ACI _____

3. Heat-related conditions

Peer _____

ACI _____

4. Sport-specific hazards

Peer _____

ACI _____

5. Weight chart

Peer _____

ACI _____

Anaphylaxis and Asthma Attacks

Objective

Demonstrate the skills necessary to use epinephrine and bronchodilators in an emergency to prevent anaphylaxis and asthma attacks, respectively.

Competencies

1. Explain the legal implication of an athletic trainer using epinephrine.

2. Demonstrate the ability to use an epinephrine injection in an emergency to prevent anaphylaxis:

   a. Identify indications for an epinephrine injection.

   b. Demonstrate verbal and nonverbal instructions necessary to properly use an epinephrine injection.

   c. Identify signs and symptoms associated with an allergic reaction to, or overdose of, epinephrine.

   d. Identify countermeasures you would take if you suspected an allergic reaction to, or overdose of, epinephrine.

   e. Demonstrate proper storage of injectable epinephrine.

   f. Demonstrate proper disposal of used injection system.

3. Demonstrate the ability to use an emergency bronchodilator inhaler to prevent asthma attacks:

   a. Identify indications for use of a bronchodilator.

   b. Demonstrate verbal and nonverbal instruction to properly use a bronchodilator inhaler.

   c. Identify signs and symptoms associated with an allergic reaction to or overdose of a bronchodilator.

   d. Identify countermeasures you would take if you suspected an allergic reaction to, or overdose of, a bronchodilator.

   e. Demonstrate proper storage of a bronchodilator.

References

Your state's medical, pharmacy, and athletic training practice acts

AAOS 1999 (pp. 438-459)

Martin and Yates 1998 (pp. 44-57)

Mastery and Demonstration

Practice and reinforce these competencies by reviewing your class notes and texts, observing peer teachers and certified/licensed professionals perform the skills, discussing the competencies with peer teachers and certified/licensed professionals, practicing alone and with a peer, and then demonstrating proficiency to a peer teacher. Finally, demonstrate your proficiency to an ACI.

Approved by (date and signature)

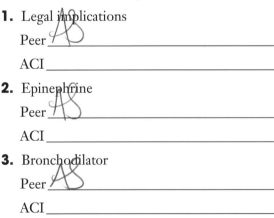

1. Legal implications

   Peer _____

   ACI _____

2. Epinephrine

   Peer _____

   ACI _____

3. Bronchodilator

   Peer _____

   ACI _____

Comments

Acute Care of Injuries and Illnesses

Poison Control Center

Objective

Demonstrate the skills necessary to report a drug overdose or poisoning to the nearest poison control center.

Competencies

1. Locate the phone number and address of the nearest poison control center.

2. Simulate reporting a drug overdose or poisoning situation, including the following:

   a. Name and location of person making the call

   b. Name and age of person who has taken the medication

   c. Name and dosage of the drug taken

   d. Time the drug was taken

   e. Signs and symptoms associated with the overdose or poisoning

   f. Vital signs of the person who has taken the medication

References

Phone book

Local hospital

Any first aid book

Mastery and Demonstration

Practice and reinforce these competencies by reviewing your class notes and texts, observing peer teachers and certified/licensed professionals perform the skills, discussing the competencies with peer teachers and certified/licensed professionals, practicing alone and with a peer, and then demonstrating proficiency to a peer teacher. Finally, demonstrate your proficiency to an ACI.

Approved by (date and signature)

1. Phone number 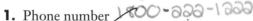 1-800-222-1222

   Peer _Dara Clausing_

   ACI _____ 9/13/10_

2. Simulation

   Peer _____

   ACI _____ 9/13/10_

Comments

Coherent + Knew what they have taken → PC

Unresponsive + don't Know → 911

→ Nausau
    Diaherra
    Rapid Heart beat
    Become unconccious
    Altered personality
  Moniter — Respiration
    heart rate

→ Put in rescue Position
  treat for
→ Shock

Level 2

Basic Skills

Athletic training students should now understand the basic operations of an athletic training clinic and be prepared to handle most emergencies that typically occur in organized athletics. Now it is time to develop and demonstrate proficiency in a wide range of psychomotor skills necessary for preventing, assessing, caring for, and rehabilitating athletic and sport injures. We call them basic skills because they are building blocks for the future, when you will integrate many of these skills in providing complete care for injured athletes.

There are 55 Level 2 modules, organized into eight groups, although your program may organize them differently.

Directed Clinical Experience

Athletic Training Clinic Student Staff

Objective

Develop and polish basic clinical skills, gain experience, and develop clinical confidence.

Competencies

1. Assist full-time and student staff in preventing, treating, and rehabilitating sports injuries. You should confine your activities to observing techniques and clinical skills you are unsure of and performing only those skills you have passed off (i.e., those that have been signed by an ACI). Thus, your activities and responsibilities will be limited to Level 1 skills at the beginning of the experience and will increase as the experience progresses. You will be assigned specific times that you are to attend, and the assignment may be to different athletic training clinics if your college has more than one or has an outreach program to other local colleges or high schools. Continue the experience until you have completed at least half of the Level 2 modules.

2. Discuss your skill development progress with an ACI.

References

Your athletic training department staff athletic trainers

Mastery and Demonstration

Obtain the signature of an ACI when you have completed this module.

Approved by (date and signature)

1. Assignment completed

   ACI: _____

2. Interview

   ACI: _____

Comments

udent Staff

M7 → Due next Tues
P18 →

body blade - changes COG

*incorporat multijoint movements
diff surfaces
change COG

Power point DAPRE
- whats the progression
- overload principle
- how to determine what a person should do the next

day

2/5

ACI: _____

Teach Level 1 Athletic Training Students

Objective

Teach Level 1 skills, assess mastery of those skills by Level 1 students, and deepen your own understanding and mastery of those skills.

Competencies

1. Peer teach at least five different Level 1 students and at least 15 Level 1 modules. This includes reviewing material with the students, offering suggestions and corrections as they practice the skills, and then assessing their mastery of the skill when appropriate. Students must practice the skills long enough that they become proficient with them before the assessment. Refer often to references and teaching aids.

2. Discuss your peer teaching experience with a faculty athletic trainer or approved clinical instructor.

References

Your athletic training department library and the references to individual Level 1 modules

Mastery and Demonstration

1. Record your peer teaching experiences in the spaces provided.

Name of Student	Module	Review Date	Assessment Date
1. Alyssa Wilkins	wrist taping		
2. alyssa wilkins	Ankle taping		
3. Katie Bultema	Ankle taping		
4. Katie Dirkse	Ankle taping		
5. Katie Dirkse	wrist taping		
6. Melissa Price	Ankle taping		
7. Melissa Price	wrist taping		
8. Eric Carlisle	wrist		
9. Eric Carlisle	ankle		
10. Kolton Reeverts	wrist		
11. Kolton Reeverts	ankle		
12. Kolton Reeverts	icebag		
13. Eric Carlse	ice bag		
14. Mackenzie Stevenson	Ankle		
15. Mackenzie Stevenson	wrist		
16. Zachery Menner	Ankle		

Module T1—Teach Level 1 Athletic Training Students (continued)

Name of Student	Module	Review Date	Assessment Date
17. *Zachary Newman*	Wrist		
18.			
19.			
20.			
21.			
22.			
23.			
24.			
25.			
26.			
27.			
28.			
29.			
30.			

2. Task completed and discussed (date)

_____

Approved by

_____

Comments

Ankle Taping, Wrapping, and Bracing

Objective

Develop and then demonstrate the ability to tape, wrap, and brace the ankle for prophylaxis or treatment of common ankle injuries.

Competencies

1. Demonstrate your ability to apply an elastic wrap for post–ankle sprain compression and support correctly, neatly, and quickly.

2. Demonstrate your ability to tape an ankle for prophylaxis correctly, neatly, and quickly.

3. Demonstrate your ability to tape an acutely sprained ankle correctly, neatly, and quickly so that the athlete can practice or compete.

4. Demonstrate your ability to properly select and apply a prophylactic ankle brace. Have your "subject" exercise for a few minutes to evaluate the method by which you attached the brace to his or her limb.

5. Demonstrate your ability to properly fit and apply an injury brace to an acutely sprained ankle so that an athlete can practice or compete. Have your subject exercise for a few minutes to evaluate your application.

References

Arnheim and Prentice 2000 (pp. 174, 186-188, 192-196, 200-204)

Perrin 1995 (pp. 18-25)

Wright and Whitehill 1991 (pp. 2:21-2:34)

Mastery and Demonstration

Practice and reinforce these competencies by reviewing your class notes and texts, observing peer teachers and certified/licensed professionals perform the skills, discussing the competencies with peer teachers and certified/licensed professionals, practicing alone and with a peer, and then demonstrating proficiency to a peer teacher. Finally, demonstrate your proficiency to an ACI.

Approved by (date and signature)

1. Elastic wrap

   Peer _____

   ACI _____

2. Prophylactic tape

   Peer _____

   ACI _____

3. Injury tape

   Peer _____

   ACI _____

4. Prophylactic brace

   Peer _____

   ACI _____

5. Injury brace

   Peer _____

   ACI _____

Comments

Knee Taping, Wrapping, and Bracing

Objective

Develop and then demonstrate the ability to tape, wrap, and brace the knee for prophylaxis or treatment of common knee injuries.

Competencies

1. Demonstrate your ability to apply elastic wraps correctly, neatly, and quickly as part of immediate care of the following two conditions:

   a. Collateral ligament sprain

   b. Hyperextension sprain

2. Demonstrate your ability to correctly, neatly, and quickly tape the knee to allow the athlete to practice or compete during the latter phases of rehabilitation of the following injuries:

   a. Medial collateral knee ligament (medial and/or lateral)

   b. Hyperextended knee

   c. Patellofemoral pain

3. Discuss the differences and similarities in the design and use of various types and brands of knee braces.

4. Demonstrate your ability to properly select and apply the following knee braces. Have your subject exercise for a few minutes to evaluate the method by which you attached the brace to his or her limb.

   a. Prophylactic brace

   b. Postinjury/surgery immobilization brace

   c. Injury brace

   d. Derotation brace _recovery_

   e. Patellar tracking brace

References

Arnheim and Prentice 2000 (pp. 175-176, 192-196, 204-208)

Perrin 1995 (pp. 48-50, 54-58)

Wright and Whitehill 1991 (pp. 2:41-2:58)

Mastery and Demonstration

Practice and reinforce these competencies by reviewing your class notes and texts, observing peer teachers and certified/licensed professionals perform the skills, discussing the competencies with peer teachers and certified/licensed professionals, practicing alone and with a peer, and then demonstrating proficiency to a peer teacher. Finally, demonstrate your proficiency to an ACI.

Approved by (date and signature)

1a. Elastic wrap—collateral ligament sprain

Peer_____

ACI_____

1b. Elastic wrap—hyperextension sprain

Peer_____

ACI_____

2a. Tape—medial collateral knee ligament

Peer_____

ACI_____

2b. Tape—hyperextended knee

Peer_____

ACI_____

2c. Tape—patellofemoral pain

Peer_____

ACI_____

3. Discussion

Peer_____

ACI_____

4a. Prophylactic brace

Peer_____

ACI_____

4b. Injury immobilizer

Peer _____

ACI _____

4c. Injury brace

Peer _____

ACI _____

4d. Derotation brace

Peer _____

ACI _____

4e. Patellar brace

Peer _____

ACI _____

Comments

Taping, Wrapping, Bracing, and Padding

Thigh and Lower Leg Taping, Wrapping, and Padding

Objective

Develop and then demonstrate the ability to tape, wrap, and pad the thigh and lower leg for prophylaxis or treatment of common thigh and lower leg injuries.

Competencies

1. Demonstrate your ability to apply elastic wraps correctly, neatly, and quickly as part of immediate care of a thigh strain.

2. Demonstrate your ability to correctly, neatly, and quickly tape the lower leg to allow the athlete to practice or compete during the latter phases of rehabilitation of the following injuries:

   a. Achilles tendon strain

   b. Medial tibial stress syndrome

3. Discuss the various types of material used to construct injury pads and show how each is used.

4. Fabricate a heat-moldable pad.

5. Demonstrate your ability to properly select and apply pads for the following injuries. Have your subject exercise for a few minutes to evaluate the method by which you attached the pad.

   a. Quadriceps contusion

   b. Shin contusion

References

Arnheim and Prentice 2000 (pp. 188-190, 192-196, 203-204)

Perrin 1995 (pp. 29-30, 38-39)

Wright and Whitehill 1991 (pp. 2:35-2:40, 2:59-2:64)

Mastery and Demonstration

Practice and reinforce these competencies by reviewing your class notes and texts, observing peer teachers and certified/licensed professionals perform the skills, discussing the competencies with peer teachers and certified/licensed professionals, practicing alone and with a peer, and then demonstrating proficiency to a peer teacher. Finally, demonstrate your proficiency to an ACI.

Approved by (date and signature)

1. Elastic wrap

   Peer _Bethany Hyde_

   ACI _____

2a. Tape—Achilles

   Peer _BH_

   ACI _____

2b. Tape—tibia

   Peer _BH_

   ACI _____

3. Discuss pad materials

   Peer _BH_

   ACI _____

4. Heat moldable

   Peer _BH_

   ACI _____

5a. Pad—quads

   Peer _BH_

   ACI _____

5b. Pad—shin

Peer _____

ACI _____

Comments

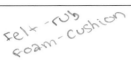

Taping, Wrapping, Bracing, and Padding

Foot Care, Taping, Wrapping, and Padding

Objective

Develop and then demonstrate the ability to care for, tape, wrap, and pad the foot for prophylaxis or treatment of common foot injuries and conditions.

Competencies

1. Demonstrate your ability to care for the following foot injuries:

use felt

  a. Blister - *Donen+ pad /Skin care*

  b. Corns and bunions - *Donen+ pad*

  c. Ingrown toenail - *Soak it. Triple Badiclue* *warm water*

Shave down when painful

2. Demonstrate your ability to correctly, neatly, and quickly tape the foot to allow the athlete to practice or compete during the latter phases of rehabilitation of the following injuries:

  a. Sprained hallux

  b. Sprained digit

  c. Longitudinal arch

  d. Heel bruise

3. Discuss the differences and similarities in the design and use of various types and brands of specialty foot pads.

4. Demonstrate your ability to properly select and apply the following foot pads. Have your subject exercise for a few minutes to evaluate the method by which you attached the pad to his or her limb.

  a. Metatarsal stress fracture

  b. Toe fracture

  c. Heel spur

  d. Heel bruise

References

Arnheim and Prentice 2000 (pp. 176-181, 192-203)

Perrin 1995 (pp. 31-37)

Wright and Whitehill 1991 (pp. 2:8-2:20)

Mastery and Demonstration

Practice and reinforce these competencies by reviewing your class notes and texts, observing peer teachers and certified/licensed professionals perform the skills, discussing the competencies with peer teachers and certified/licensed professionals, practicing alone and with a peer, and then demonstrating proficiency to a peer teacher. Finally, demonstrate your proficiency to an ACI.

Approved by (date and signature)

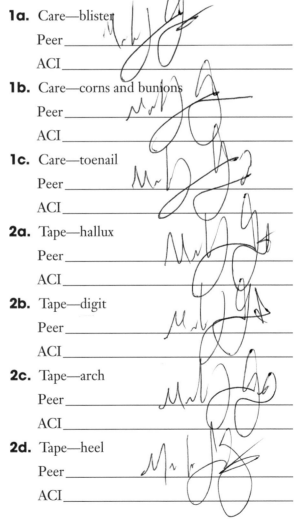

1a. Care—blister

Peer _____

ACI _____

1b. Care—corns and bunions

Peer _____

ACI _____

1c. Care—toenail

Peer _____

ACI _____

2a. Tape—hallux

Peer _____

ACI _____

2b. Tape—digit

Peer _____

ACI _____

2c. Tape—arch

Peer _____

ACI _____

2d. Tape—heel

Peer _____

ACI _____

3. Discussion 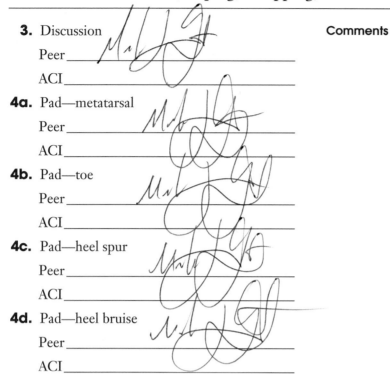   Comments

Peer

ACI

4a. Pad—metatarsal

Peer

ACI

4b. Pad—toe

Peer

ACI

4c. Pad—heel spur

Peer

ACI

4d. Pad—heel bruise

Peer

ACI

Hip and Abdomen Taping, Wrapping, and Bracing

Objective

Develop and then demonstrate the ability to tape and wrap the hip and abdomen for prophylaxis or treatment of common hip and abdomen injuries.

Competencies

1. Demonstrate your ability to apply elastic wraps correctly, neatly, and quickly as part of immediate care of the following two conditions:

   a. Groin strain—adductors

   b. Groin strain—flexors

2. Demonstrate your ability to correctly, neatly, and quickly tape the hip/abdomen to allow the athlete to practice or compete during the latter phases of rehabilitation of a hip pointer.

3. Demonstrate your ability to properly select and apply a brace for a lumbosacral sprain. Have your subject exercise for a few minutes to evaluate the method by which you attached the brace to his or her limb.

References

Arnheim and Prentice 2000 (pp. 188, 192-196)

Perrin 1995 (pp. 64-70)

Wright and Whitehill 1991 (pp. 3:6-3:7)

Mastery and Demonstration

Practice and reinforce these competencies by reviewing your class notes and texts, observing peer teachers and certified/licensed professionals perform the skills, discussing the competencies with peer teachers and certified/licensed professionals, practicing alone and with a peer, and then demonstrating proficiency to a peer teacher. Finally, demonstrate your proficiency to an ACI.

Approved by (date and signature)

1a. Groin—adduct

Peer _Michael Etales_

ACI _____

1b. Groin—flexors

Peer _____ m S _____

ACI _____

2. Hip pointer pad

Peer _____ m S _____

ACI _____

3. Lumbosacral sprain

Peer _____ m S _____

ACI _____

Comments

Taping, Wrapping, Bracing, and Padding

Shoulder Taping, Wrapping, and Bracing

Objective

Develop and then demonstrate the ability to tape, wrap, and brace the shoulder for prophylaxis or treatment of common shoulder injuries.

Competencies

1. Demonstrate your ability to apply the three following bandages to the shoulder correctly, neatly, and quickly as part of immediate care of a shoulder injury:

   a. Shoulder sling (cloth)

   b. Shoulder sling (elastic wraps)

   c. Shoulder spica (elastic wraps)

2. Demonstrate your ability to correctly, neatly, and quickly tape the shoulder/chest to allow the athlete to practice or compete during the latter phases of rehabilitation of:

   a. Acromioclavicular (AC) sprain

   b. Sternoclavicular (SC) sprain

3. Discuss the differences and similarities in the design and use of various types and brands of shoulder braces.

4. Demonstrate your ability to properly select and apply the following shoulder pads/braces. Have your subject exercise for a few minutes to evaluate the method by which you attached the brace to his or her limb.

   a. Shoulder harness

   b. Shoulder pads

   c. AC pad

   d. SC pad

References

Arnheim and Prentice 2000 (pp. 188, 190-196)

Perrin 1995 (pp. 76-83)

Wright and Whitehill 1991 (pp. 4:16-4:29)

Mastery and Demonstration

Practice and reinforce these competencies by reviewing your class notes and texts, observing peer teachers and certified/licensed professionals perform the skills, discussing the competencies with peer teachers and certified/licensed professionals, practicing alone and with a peer, and then demonstrating proficiency to a peer teacher. Finally, demonstrate your proficiency to an ACI.

Approved by (date and signature)

1a. Sling—cloth

Peer _Bethany Hyde_

ACI _Cyril Kamde_

1b. Sling—elastic

Peer _BH_

ACI _Cyril Kamde_

1c. Spica

Peer _BH_

ACI _Cyril Kamde_

2a. AC tape

Peer _____

ACI _____

2b. SC tape

Peer _____

ACI _____

3. Discussion

Peer _____

ACI _____

4a. Harness

Peer _____

ACI _____

Module C6—Shoulder Taping, Wrapping, and Bracing (continued)

4b. Shoulder pads

Peer _____

ACI _____

4c. AC pad

Peer _____

ACI _____

4d. SC pad

Peer _____

ACI _____

Comments

Taping, Wrapping, Bracing, and Padding

Elbow-to-Wrist Taping, Wrapping, and Bracing

Objective

Develop and then demonstrate the ability to tape, wrap, and brace the elbow, forearm, and wrist for prophylaxis or treatment of common elbow, forearm, and wrist injuries.

Competencies

1. Demonstrate your ability to apply elastic wraps correctly, neatly, and quickly as part of immediate care of an elbow contusion.

2. Demonstrate your ability to apply elastic or cloth wraps to the wrist correctly, neatly, and quickly to allow an athlete with a sprained wrist to practice or compete during the latter phases of rehabilitation in the following two sports:

   a. Football

   b. Gymnastics

3. Demonstrate your ability to apply a double-friction blister pad to the wrist of a gymnast with severe blisters to allow him or her to compete on rings or bars.

4. Demonstrate your ability to correctly, neatly, and quickly tape the elbow/arm/wrist to allow the athlete to practice or compete during the latter phases of rehabilitation of the following injuries:

   a. Elbow hyperextension

   b. Collateral ligament sprain

   c. Forearm splints

   d. Wrist flexor strain

   e. Wrist extensor strain

5. Discuss the differences and similarities in the design and use of various types and brands of elbow braces.

6. Demonstrate your ability to properly select and apply the following brace and pad. Have your subject exercise for a few minutes to evaluate the method by which you attached the brace to his or her limb.

   a. Epicondylitis

   b. Olecranon bursa contusion using closed cell foam

References

Arnheim and Prentice 2000 (pp. 176, 189, 192-196, 207)

Perrin 1995 (pp. 90-95, 104-113)

Wright and Whitehill 1991 (pp. 4:16-4:29)

Mastery and Demonstration

Practice and reinforce these competencies by reviewing your class notes and texts, observing peer teachers and certified/licensed professionals perform the skills, discussing the competencies with peer teachers and certified/licensed professionals, practicing alone and with a peer, and then demonstrating proficiency to a peer teacher. Finally, demonstrate your proficiency to an ACI.

Approved by (date and signature)

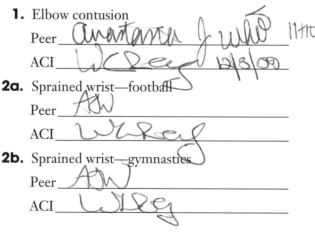

1. Elbow contusion

   Peer _____

   ACI _____

2a. Sprained wrist—football

   Peer _____

   ACI _____

2b. Sprained wrist—gymnastics

   Peer _____

   ACI _____

3. Wrist—friction blister

Peer _____

ACI _____

Comments

Vball

5

4a. Elbow hyperextension

Peer _____

ACI _____

4b. Collateral ligament sprain

Peer _____

ACI _____

4c. Forearm splints

Peer _____

ACI _____

4d. Wrist—flexor

Peer _____

ACI _____

4e. Wrist—extensor

Peer _____

ACI _____

5. Discussion

Peer _____

ACI _____

6a. Epicondylitis

Peer _____

ACI _____

6b. Bursa

Peer _____

ACI _____

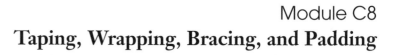
mallet —
boot —

Taping, Wrapping, Bracing, and Padding

Hand and Finger Taping and Wrapping

Objective

Develop and then demonstrate the ability to tape and wrap the hand and fingers for prophylaxis or treatment of common hand and finger injuries.

Competencies

1. Demonstrate your ability to tape a sprained finger correctly, neatly, and quickly as part of immediate care.

2. Demonstrate your ability to correctly, neatly, and quickly tape the hand/fingers to allow the athlete to practice or compete during the latter phases of rehabilitation of the following injuries:

   a. Hand contusion

   b. Thumb sprain

   c. Proximal interphalangeal (PIP) sprain

   d. Distal interphalangeal (DIP) sprain

   e. Boutonniere

   f. Finger dislocation

   g. Finger hyperextension

   h. Mallet finger

References

Arnheim and Prentice 2000 (pp. 190-196, 209-210)

Perrin 1995 (pp. 112-113)

Wright and Whitehill 1991 (pp. 4:30-4:44)

Mastery and Demonstration

Practice and reinforce these competencies by reviewing your class notes and texts, observing peer teachers and certified/licensed professionals perform the skills, discussing the competencies with peer teachers and certified/licensed professionals, practicing alone and with a peer, and then demonstrating proficiency to a peer teacher. Finally, demonstrate your proficiency to an ACI.

Approved by (date and signature)

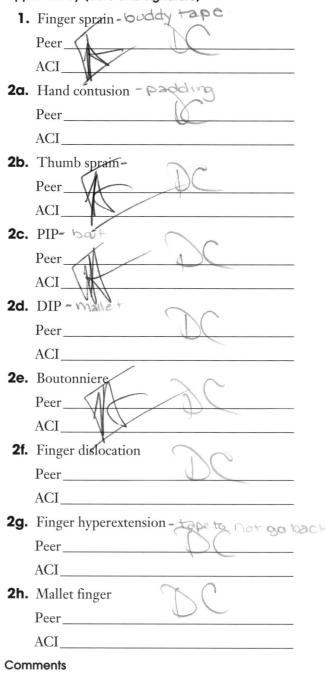

1. Finger sprain – *buddy tape*

Peer _____

ACI _____

2a. Hand contusion – *padding*

Peer _____

ACI _____

2b. Thumb sprain –

Peer _____

ACI _____

2c. PIP – *bat*

Peer _____

ACI _____

2d. DIP – *mallet*

Peer _____

ACI _____

2e. Boutonniere

Peer _____

ACI _____

2f. Finger dislocation

Peer _____

ACI _____

2g. Finger hyperextension – *tape to not go back*

Peer _____

ACI _____

2h. Mallet finger

Peer _____

ACI _____

Comments

Head and Neck Padding and Bracing

Objective

Develop and then demonstrate the ability to pad and brace the head and neck for prophylaxis or treatment of common head and neck injuries.

Competencies

1. Fit an off-the-shelf mouthpiece or manufacture a custom mouthpiece (the type used by your athletic department).

2. Manufacture or fit a customized face mask to a basketball player to protect a facial or nose fracture.

3. Fit a neck roll to prevent a neck hyperextension injury.

4. Fit a cervical collar for emergency management of a neck injury.

References

Anderson, Hall, and Martin 2000 (pp. 43-48)

Arnheim and Prentice 2000 (p. 164)

Mastery and Demonstration

Practice and reinforce these competencies by reviewing your class notes and texts, observing peer teachers and certified/licensed professionals perform the skills, discussing the competencies with peer teachers and certified/licensed professionals, practicing alone and with a peer, and then demonstrating proficiency to a peer teacher. Finally, demonstrate your proficiency to an ACI.

Approved by (date and signature)

1. Mouthpiece

   Peer _____

   ACI _____

2. Face mask

   Peer _____

   ACI _____

3. Neck roll

   Peer _____

   ACI _____

4. Collar

   Peer _____

   ACI _____

Comments

Anthropometric Measurements and Screening Procedures

Objective

Develop the skills necessary to accurately perform anthropometric measurement techniques and other appropriate examination and screening procedures.

Competencies

1. Define "measurement reliability" and "measurement validity."

2. Measure the following on at least five people on two different days. Record your results.
   a. Height
   b. Weight
   c. Blood pressure
   d. Pulse
   e. Limb girth
   f. Limb length
   g. Vision, using a Snellen eye chart
   h. Body composition, using a manual skinfold caliper and appropriate formulas

3. Discuss the results of the measurements in Item 2, including how they relate to measurement reliability and validity.

References

An exercise physiology text

Mastery and Demonstration

Practice and reinforce these competencies by reviewing your class notes and texts, observing peer teachers and certified/licensed professionals perform the skills, discussing the competencies with peer teachers and certified/licensed professionals, practicing alone and with a peer, and then demonstrating proficiency to a peer teacher. Finally, demonstrate your proficiency to an ACI.

www. linear-software .com/online.html

Approved by (date and signature)

1. Definitions

   Peer _____

   ACI _____

2. Measurements

   Peer _____

   ACI _____

3. Discussion

   Peer _____

   ACI _____

Comments

HW
Take 5 BP
record #s

Ticep + Thigh all on a person

BP
140/90 → High BP

Protective Equipment Fitting

Objective

Develop and demonstrate the skills necessary to properly select and fit protective athletic equipment.

Competencies

1. Select and fit the following protective equipment to at least two different athletes:

    a. Protective helmet and head gear for football, ice hockey, and lacrosse

    b. Football and hockey shoulder pads

    c. Footwear for physical activity

    d. Rib brace/guard

References

Anderson, Hall, and Martin 2000 (pp. 31-56)

Arnheim and Prentice 2000 (pp. 158-184)

Mastery and Demonstration

Practice and reinforce these competencies by reviewing your class notes and texts, observing peer teachers and certified/licensed professionals perform the skills, discussing the competencies with peer teachers and certified/licensed professionals, practicing alone and with a peer, and then demonstrating proficiency to a peer teacher. Finally, demonstrate your proficiency to an ACI.

Approved by (date and signature)

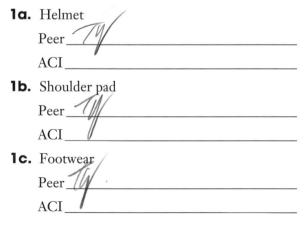

1a. Helmet

    Peer _____

    ACI _____

1b. Shoulder pad

    Peer _____

    ACI _____

1c. Footwear

    Peer _____

    ACI _____

1d. Rib brace/guard

    Peer _____

    ACI _____

Comments

Developing Flexibility

Objective

Develop and demonstrate the skills necessary to properly develop flexibility.

Competencies

1. Instruct and demonstrate exercises to develop flexibility for the following:

  a. Cervical region

  b. Shoulder girdle

  c. Elbow

  d. Wrist

  e. Hand and fingers

  f. Lumbar region

  g. Hip and pelvis

  h. Knee

  i. Lower leg

  j. Ankle

  k. Foot and toes

References

Allsen, Harrison, and Vance 1997 (pp. 190-215)

Hillman 2000 (pp. 153-155)

Mastery and Demonstration

Practice and reinforce these competencies by reviewing your class notes and texts, observing peer teachers and certified/licensed professionals perform the skills, discussing the competencies with peer teachers and certified/licensed professionals, practicing alone and with a peer, and then demonstrating proficiency to a peer teacher. Finally, demonstrate your proficiency to an ACI.

Approved by (date and signature)

1a. Cervical region

  Peer_____

  ACI_____

1b. Shoulder girdle

  Peer_____

  ACI_____

1c. Elbow

  Peer_____

  ACI_____

1d. Wrist

  Peer_____

  ACI_____

1e. Hand/fingers

  Peer_____

  ACI_____

1f. Lumbar region

  Peer_____

  ACI_____

1g. Hip/pelvis

  Peer_____

  ACI_____

1h. Knee

  Peer_____

  ACI_____

1i. Lower leg

  Peer_____

  ACI_____

1j. Ankle

  Peer_____

  ACI_____

1k. Foot/toes   **Comments**

Peer_____

ACI_____

Strength Training

Objective

Develop and demonstrate the skills necessary to teach proper strength-training techniques.

Competencies

1. Instruct and demonstrate proper lifting technique for the following:
   a. Parallel squat
   b. Heel raises
   c. Power clean
   d. Bench press
   e. Shoulder press
   f. Dead lift
   g. Arm curl
   h. Triceps extension
   i. Knee curl (flexion)
   j. Knee extension
   k. Leg press

2. Instruct and demonstrate the proper spotting technique for the following:
   a. Parallel squat
   b. Shoulder press
   c. Dead lift
   d. Bench press
   e. Power clean

References

Allsen, Harrison, and Vance 1997 (pp. 145-179)

Hillman 2000 (pp. 128-130, 141-159)

Merten and Potteiger 1991

Mastery and Demonstration

Practice and reinforce these competencies by reviewing your class notes and texts, observing peer teachers and certified/licensed professionals perform the skills, discussing the competencies with peer teachers and certified/licensed professionals, practicing alone and with a peer, and then demonstrating proficiency to a peer teacher. Finally, demonstrate your proficiency to an ACI.

Approved by (date and signature)

1a. Parallel squat
Peer _____
ACI _____

1b. Heel raises
Peer _____
ACI _____

1c. Power clean
Peer _____
ACI _____

1d. Bench press
Peer _____
ACI _____

1e. Shoulder press
Peer _____
ACI _____

1f. Dead lift
Peer _____
ACI _____

1g. Arm curl
Peer _____
ACI _____

1h. Triceps extension
Peer _____
ACI _____

1i. Knee curl (flexion)

Peer _____

ACI _____

1j. Knee extension

Peer _____

ACI _____

1k. Leg press

Peer _____

ACI _____

2a. Spotting parallel squat

Peer _____

ACI _____

2b. Spotting shoulder press

Peer _____

ACI _____

2c. Spotting dead lift

Peer _____

ACI _____

2d. Spotting bench press

Peer _____

ACI _____

2e. Spotting power clean

Peer _____

ACI _____

Comments

General Medical Assessment

Objective

Demonstrate your ability to assess a person's general medical status.

Competencies

1. Take a basic medical history that includes at least the following components:
   a. Previous medical history
   b. Previous surgical history
   c. Pertinent family medical history
   d. Current medication history
   e. Relevant social history
   f. Chief medical complaint

2. Measure body temperature via the following methods. Tell how each relates to core temperature and to each other.
   a. Oral temperature
   b. Axillary temperature
   c. Tympanic temperature

3. Measure the following vital signs:
   a. Blood pressure
   b. Pulse (rate and quality)
   c. Respiration (rate and quality)

4. Palpate the four abdominal quadrants. Tell how you would know if the patient experienced pain or guarding and rigidity during your palpation. What medical conditions do each of these signs indicate?

5. Identify the following with a stethoscope:
   a. Normal breath sounds
   b. Normal heart sounds
   c. Normal bowel sounds

6. Identify pathological breathing patterns associated with the following respiratory conditions. Tell how these can be used to make a differential assessment of the following respiratory conditions:
   a. Apnea
   b. Tachypnea
   c. Hyperventilation
   d. Bradypnea
   e. Dyspnea
   f. Obstructed airway

7. Use an otoscope to examine the nose and the outer and middle ear.

8. Measure urine values with Chemstrips (dipsticks). What are normal values, and what do abnormal values indicate?

References

Team physician

ACI

Mastery and Demonstration

Practice and reinforce these competencies by reviewing your class notes and texts, observing peer teachers and certified/licensed professionals perform the skills, discussing the competencies with peer teachers and certified/licensed professionals, practicing alone and with a peer, and then demonstrating proficiency to a peer teacher. Finally, demonstrate your proficiency to an ACI.

Approved by (date and signature)

1. General history

Peer _____

ACI _____

2. Temperature

Peer _____

ACI _____

Module E1—General Medical Assessment (continued)

3. Vital signs

Peer _____

ACI _____

4. Palpate

Peer _____

ACI _____

5. Stethoscope

Peer _____

ACI _____

6. Breathing patterns

Peer _____

ACI _____

7. Otoscope

Peer _____

ACI _____

8. Urine

Peer _____

ACI _____

Comments

LEVEL 2

Basic Assessment and Evaluation

Postural Assessment

Objective

Develop and demonstrate the skills necessary to properly assess and evaluate normal and abnormal posture.

Competencies

1. Perform a postural assessment of the following:
   a. Cervical spine and head
   b. Shoulder
   c. Lumbothoracic region
   d. Hip and pelvis
   e. Knee
   f. Ankle, foot, and toes

2. Identify each of the following postural deviations and tell how they can predispose an athlete to injury.
   a. Kyphosis
   b. Lordosis
   c. Scoliosis
   d. Pelvic obliquity
   e. Tibial torsion
   f. Hip anteversion and retroversion
   g. Genu valgum, varum, and recurvatum
   h. Rearfoot valgus and varus
   i. Forefoot valgus and varus
   j. Pes cavus and planus
   k. Foot and toe posture

3. Identify the characteristics of each of the following body types. Name three athletes at your institution who would be classified in each category.
   a. Endomorph
   b. Ectomorph
   c. Mesomorph

Funtion – U
Anatomical – ASIS

References

Exercise physiology text

Anderson, Hall, and Martin 2000 (pp. 233, 308, 418, 464, 520)

Arnheim and Prentice 2000 (pp. 234-235, 707-709)

Magee 1997 (pp. 697-725)

Starkey and Ryan 2002 (pp. 52-85)

Mastery and Demonstration

Practice and reinforce these competencies by reviewing your class notes and texts, observing peer teachers and certified/licensed professionals perform the skills, discussing the competencies with peer teachers and certified/licensed professionals, practicing alone and with a peer, and then demonstrating proficiency to a peer teacher. Finally, demonstrate your proficiency to an ACI.

Approved by (date and signature)

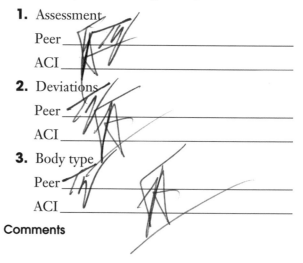

1. Assessment
   Peer _____
   ACI _____

2. Deviations
   Peer _____
   ACI _____

3. Body type
   Peer _____
   ACI _____

Comments

Philip Tayl 5/5

Basic Assessment and Evaluation

Neurological Assessment

Objective

Develop and demonstrate the skills necessary to properly identify and assess the following neurological structures and functions.

Competencies

1. Identify and assess the following:

a. Cranial nerves

b. Dermatomes

c. Myotomes

d. Deep tendon reflexes

e. Pathological reflexes

References

Anderson, Hall, and Martin 2000 (pp. 79, 182, 245, 351, 477, 525, 673)

Arnheim and Prentice 2000 (pp. 318-319, 721-722)

Starkey and Ryan 2002 (pp. 1-22)

Mastery and Demonstration

Practice and reinforce these competencies by reviewing your class notes and texts, observing peer teachers and certified/licensed professionals perform the skills, discussing the competencies with peer teachers and certified/licensed professionals, practicing alone and with a peer, and then demonstrating proficiency to a peer teacher. Finally, demonstrate your proficiency to an ACI.

Approved by (date and signature)

1a. Cranial

Peer _____

ACI _____

1b. Dermatomes

Peer _____

ACI _____

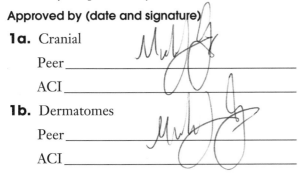

1c. Myotomes

Peer _____

ACI _____

1d. Deep tendon reflexes

Peer _____

ACI _____

1e. Pathological reflexes

Peer _____

ACI _____

Comments

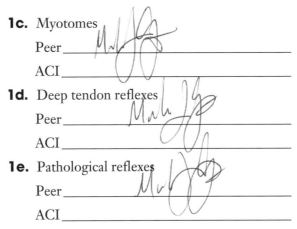

Palpation

Objective

Develop and demonstrate the skills necessary to palpate anatomical structures.

Competencies

1. Identify the following by palpation:

    a. Bony landmarks of the head, trunk, spine, scapula, and extremities

    b. Soft tissue structures of the head, trunk, spine, and extremities

    c. Abdominal and thoracic structures

    d. Primary neurological and circulatory structures

References

Anderson, Hall, and Martin 2000 (numerous, see index)

Arnheim and Prentice 2000 (numerous, see index)

Shultz, Houglum, and Perrin 2000 (pp. 26-28)

Starkey and Ryan 2002 (pp. 1-22)

Mastery and Demonstration

Practice and reinforce these competencies by reviewing your class notes and texts, observing peer teachers and certified/licensed professionals perform the skills, discussing the competencies with peer teachers and certified/licensed professionals, practicing alone and with a peer, and then demonstrating proficiency to a peer teacher. Finally, demonstrate your proficiency to an ACI.

Approved by (date and signature)

1a. Bony landmarks

    Peer_____

    ACI_____

1b. Soft tissue

    Peer_____

    ACI_____

1c. Abdominal/thoracic

    Peer_____

    ACI_____

1d. Neurological/circulatory

    Peer_____

    ACI_____

Comments

Assessing Range of Motion

Objective

Develop and demonstrate the skills necessary to assess range of motion (ROM).

Competencies

1. Qualitatively assess active, passive, and resistive ROM of the following:

    a. Temporomandibular joint (TMJ)

    b. Cervical spine

    c. Shoulder

    d. Elbow

    e. Wrist and hand

    f. Thumb and fingers

    g. Hip

    h. Lumbar spine

    i. Thoracic spine

    j. Knee

    k. Ankle

    l. Foot and toes

References

Arnheim and Prentice 2000 (pp. 76-87)

Houglum 2001 (pp.120-150)

Prentice 1999 (pp. 62-72)

Starkey and Ryan 2002 (pp. 1-22)

Mastery and Demonstration

Practice and reinforce these competencies by reviewing your class notes and texts, observing peer teachers and certified/licensed professionals perform the skills, discussing the competencies with peer teachers and certified/licensed professionals, practicing alone and with a peer, and then demonstrating proficiency to a peer teacher. Finally, demonstrate your proficiency to an ACI.

Approved by (date and signature)

1a. TMJ

Peer_____

ACI_____

1b. Cervical spine

Peer_____

ACI_____

1c. Shoulder

Peer_____

ACI_____

1d. Elbow

Peer_____

ACI_____

1e. Wrist and hand

Peer_____

ACI_____

1f. Thumb and fingers

Peer_____

ACI_____

1g. Hip

Peer_____

ACI_____

1h. Lumbar spine

Peer_____

ACI_____

1i. Thoracic spine

Peer_____

ACI_____

1j. Knee

    Peer_____

    ACI_____

1k. Ankle

    Peer_____

    ACI_____

1l. Foot and toes

    Peer_____

    ACI_____

Comments

Physical Performance Measurements

Objective

Develop and demonstrate the skills necessary to properly measure selected elements of physical performance.

Competencies

1. Perform and interpret repetition maximum tests to measure the strength of the following:
   a. Elbow flexors
   b. Leg (leg press or squat)

2. Perform and interpret isokinetic tests to measure the strength of the following:
   a. Knee (extensors)
   b. Shoulder (press)

3. Perform and interpret isometric tests for the following:
   a. Ankle
   b. Foot and toes
   c. Knee
   d. Hip
   e. Trunk and torso
   f. Shoulder
   g. Elbow
   h. Wrist
   i. Hand and fingers

4. Perform and interpret the following tests:
   a. Upper body strength test
   b. Lower body strength test
   c. Upper body power test
   d. Lower body power test
   e. Upper body muscular endurance test
   f. Lower body muscular endurance test
   g. Agility
   h. Speed

References

Hillman 2000 (pp. 118-159)

Starkey and Ryan 2002 (pp. 1-22)

Mastery and Demonstration

Practice and reinforce these competencies by reviewing your class notes and texts, observing peer teachers and certified/licensed professionals perform the skills, discussing the competencies with peer teachers and certified/licensed professionals, practicing alone and with a peer, and then demonstrating proficiency to a peer teacher. Finally, demonstrate your proficiency to an ACI.

Approved by (date and signature)

1. Repetition maximum tests

   Peer _____

   ACI _____

2. Isokinetic tests

   Peer _____

   ACI _____

3. Isometric tests

   Peer _____

   ACI _____

4a. Strength—upper body

   Peer _____

   ACI _____

4b. Strength—lower body

   Peer _____

   ACI _____

4c. Power—upper body

   Peer _____

   ACI _____

4d. Power—lower body

     Peer _____

     ACI _____

4e. Endurance—upper body

     Peer _____

     ACI _____

4f. Endurance—lower body

     Peer _____

     ACI _____

4g. Agility

     Peer _____

     ACI _____

4h. Speed

     Peer _____

     ACI _____

Comments

Basic Pharmacology and Nutrition

Medication Resources

Objective

Develop and demonstrate the skills necessary to properly use the *Physician's Desk Reference* (PDR), *Drug Facts and Comparisons*, or on-line resources for obtaining information on medications related to athletic training.

Competencies *epocrates*

1. Use the ~~PDR~~ or another drug reference to search for information on the medications commonly prescribed to athletes and others involved in physical activity and to identify the following information:

   (a.) Generic and brand names

   (b) Indications for use

   (c) Contraindications

   (d) Warnings

   (e.) Dosing

   f. Other notes (e.g., banned substance)

   (g.) Side (adverse) effects

References

PDR, published yearly

Hillman 2000 (p. 171)

Drug Facts and Comparisons, published yearly

Mastery and Demonstration

Practice and reinforce these competencies by reviewing your class notes and texts, observing peer teachers and certified/licensed professionals perform the skills, discussing the competencies with peer teachers and certified/licensed professionals, practicing alone and with a peer, and then demonstrating proficiency to a peer teacher. Finally, demonstrate your proficiency to an ACI.

Approved by (date and signature)

1. PDR

   Peer _____

   ACI _____

Comments

Ibpro
Tylenol
Asprin
Mobic
Celebrex
Aleve
Sudorine/Sudopedrine
Cephalexin
Amoxicillian
Guiaiffen
Codine
Vicodin
Perchocet

Define & explain

Bioavailability
Half-life
bioequivalence

Medication Policies and Procedures

Objective

Demonstrate an understanding of your university's medication policies and procedures, including tracking medications dispensed to athletes.

Competencies

1. Explain the main points of your state's laws governing prescriptions and dispensing prescription and over-the-counter (OTC) medications.

2. Obtain a copy of the medication section of your institution's athletic training policies and procedures manual. Discuss these policies, including the following:

   a. The established protocols for use of OTC medications.

   b. The types of OTC medications to be used according to the physical ailment.

   c. How to identify the precautions, expiration date, lot number, and dosage of medications as provided on the package and individual dose packets.

   d. Verbal and written instructions given to patients when administering OTC medication to them.

   e. Recording and documenting required when administering OTC medication.

3. Document the tracking of medications by recording the following information about the medication:

   a. Name of athlete

   b. Date medication given

   c. Name of medication

   d. Manufacturer

   e. Amount

   f. Dosage

   g. Lot number

   h. Expiration date

+Make Spread Sheet

References

Your state's medical, pharmacy, and athletic training practice acts

Martin and Yates 1998 (pp. 5-12)

Hillman 2000 (pp. 163-203)

Mastery and Demonstration

Practice and reinforce these competencies by reviewing your class notes and texts, observing peer teachers and certified/licensed professionals perform the skills, discussing the competencies with peer teachers and certified/licensed professionals, practicing alone and with a peer, and then demonstrating proficiency to a peer teacher. Finally, demonstrate your proficiency to an ACI.

Approved by (date and signature)

1. Legal implications

Peer _____

ACI _____

2. Policy and procedures

Peer _____

ACI _____

3. Documentation

Peer _____

ACI _____

Comments

Basic Performance Nutrition

Objective

Demonstrate a knowledge of basic nutritional guidelines for athletes.

Competencies

1. Discuss the Recommended Daily Allowances (RDA) nutritional food pyramid and demonstrate how you would use it in counseling athletes about appropriate nutrition.

2. Access the following nutritional intake values for a male and a female athlete:
   a. RDA or equivalency
   b. Protein intake
   c. Fat intake
   d. Carbohydrate intake
   e. Vitamin intake
   f. Mineral intake
   g. Fluid intake

3. Calculate the basal metabolic rate (BMR) of energy expenditure for the following:
   a. Female gymnast
   b. Football linebacker
   c. Distance swimmer

4. Using standard resources, calculate the energy expenditure and optimal caloric intake of the athletes in Item 3.

5. Demonstrate your ability to access current nutritional guidelines for the following:
   a. Preparticipation meal
   b. Weight loss
   c. Weight gain
   d. Fluid replacement

6. Using the resources in Item 1, discuss nutritional guidelines you would recommend to athletes for each of the situations listed in Item 3.

References

Allsen, Harrison, and Vance 1997 (pp. 45-70)

AAOS 1999 (pp. 602-629)

Hillman 2000 (pp. 313-330)

Mastery and Demonstration

Practice and reinforce these competencies by reviewing your class notes and texts, observing peer teachers and certified/licensed professionals perform the skills, discussing the competencies with peer teachers and certified/licensed professionals, practicing alone and with a peer, and then demonstrating proficiency to a peer teacher. Finally, demonstrate your proficiency to an ACI.

Approved by (date and signature)

1. Food pyramid

   Peer_____

   ACI_____

2. Intake values

   Peer_____

   ACI_____

3. BMR

   Peer_____

   ACI_____

4. Energy expenditure and intake

   Peer_____

   ACI_____

5. Access nutritional guidelines

   Peer_____

   ACI_____

6. Recommend nutritional guidelines   **Comments**

Peer _____

ACI _____

Basic Pharmacology and Nutrition

Eating Disorders

Objective

Demonstrate a knowledge of basic eating disorders and an ability to intervene with athletes who suffer from such disorders.

Competencies

1. Identify the common signs and symptoms of the following eating disorders:
   a. Anorexia
   b. Bulimia
   c. Obesity

2. Simulate intervention with an athlete who has the signs and symptoms of disordered eating.

3. Identify proper referral sources for disordered eating.

References

AAOS 1999 (pp. 602-629)

Anderson, Hall, and Martin 2000 (pp. 609-614)

Arnheim and Prentice 2000 (pp. 134-135)

Pfeiffer and Mangus, 1998 (pp. 57-72, 315-322)

Shultz, Houglum, and Perrin 2000 (pp. 437-439)

Mastery and Demonstration

Practice and reinforce these competencies by reviewing your class notes and texts, observing peer teachers and certified/licensed professionals perform the skills, discussing the competencies with peer teachers and certified/licensed professionals, practicing alone and with a peer, and then demonstrating proficiency to a peer teacher. Finally, demonstrate your proficiency to an ACI.

Approved by (date and signature)

1a. Anorexia

Peer_____

ACI_____

1b. Bulimia

Peer_____

ACI_____

1c. Obesity

Peer_____

ACI_____

2. Intervention

Peer_____

ACI_____

3. Referral

Peer_____

ACI_____

Comments

Whirlpool

Objective

Develop and demonstrate the skills necessary to properly use a whirlpool during sport injury rehabilitation.

Competencies

1. Define a whirlpool and briefly explain the following:

   a. Effects

   b. Advantages

   c. Disadvantages

   d. Indications

   e. Contraindications

   f. Precautions

2. Demonstrate and explain the following in relation to using a whirlpool to treat an upper extremity injury, a lower extremity injury, and general soreness:

   a. Preapplication procedures, including re-evaluating the injury, evaluating the previous treatment, setting/evaluating goals, selecting the proper modality, and preparing the modality and patient.

   b. Application procedures, including turn on, adjustments, dosage, duration, and frequency of application.

   c. Postapplication procedures, including patient and equipment cleanup, instructions to patient, scheduling next appointment.

3. Demonstrate and explain maintenance and simple repair procedures for whirlpools.

4. Demonstrate proper recording of these treatments on athletic training clinic forms.

References

Denegar 2000 (pp. 113-118)

Prentice 1999b (pp. 173-178, 190-192)

Starkey 1999 (pp. 142-147)

Mastery and Demonstration

Practice and reinforce these competencies by reviewing your class notes and texts, observing peer teachers and certified/licensed professionals perform the skills, discussing the competencies with peer teachers and certified/licensed professionals, practicing alone and with a peer, and then demonstrating proficiency to a peer teacher. Finally, demonstrate your proficiency to an ACI.

Approved by (date and signature)

1. Background

Peer _____

ACI _____

2. Application

Peer _____

ACI _____

3. Maintenance

Peer _____

ACI _____

4. Recording

Peer _____

ACI _____

Comments

LEVEL 2

Moist Hot Packs

Objective

Develop and demonstrate the skills necessary to properly use moist hot packs during sport injury rehabilitation.

Competencies

1. Define a hot pack and briefly explain the following:

  a. Effects

  b. Advantages

  c. Disadvantages

  d. Indications

  e. Contraindications

  f. Precautions

2. Demonstrate and explain the following in relation to using a moist hot pack for treating patellar tendinitis and neck soreness:

  a. Preapplication procedures, including re-evaluating the injury, evaluating results of previous treatment, setting and evaluating goals, selecting proper modality, and preparing the modality and patient.

  b. Application procedures, including turn on, adjustments, dosage, duration, and frequency of application.

  c. Postapplication procedures, including patient and equipment cleanup, instructions to the patient, and scheduling the next appointment.

3. Demonstrate and explain maintenance and simple repair procedures for moist hot packs.

4. Demonstrate proper recording of these treatments on athletic training clinic forms.

References

Denegar 2000 (pp. 113-118)

Prentice 1999b (pp. 173-178, 193-194)

Starkey 1999 (pp. 149-151)

Mastery and Demonstration

Practice and reinforce these competencies by reviewing your class notes and texts, observing peer teachers and certified/licensed professionals perform the skills, discussing the competencies with peer teachers and certified/licensed professionals, practicing alone and with a peer, and then demonstrating proficiency to a peer teacher. Finally, demonstrate your proficiency to an ACI.

Approved by (date and signature)

1. Background

  Peer

  ACI

2. Application

  Peer

  ACI

3. Maintenance

  Peer

  ACI

4. Recording

  Peer

  ACI

Comments

73

LEVEL 2

Module G3
Therapeutic Modalities

Paraffin Bath

Objective

Develop and demonstrate the skills necessary to properly use a paraffin bath during sport injury rehabilitation.

Competencies

1. Define a paraffin bath and briefly explain the following:

    a. Effects

    b. Advantages

    c. Disadvantages

    d. Indications

    e. Contraindications

    f. Precautions

2. Demonstrate and explain the following in relation to using a paraffin bath for treating a hand injury:

    a. Preapplication procedures, including re-evaluating the injury, evaluating results of previous treatment, setting and evaluating goals, selecting proper modality, and preparing the modality and patient.

    b. Application procedures, including turn on, adjustments, dosage, duration, and frequency of application.

    c. Postapplication procedures, including patient and equipment cleanup, instructions to patient, and scheduling next appointment.

3. Demonstrate and explain maintenance and simple repair procedures for paraffin baths.

4. Demonstrate proper recording of these treatments on athletic training clinic forms.

References

Denegar 2000 (pp. 113-118)

Prentice 1999b (pp. 173-178, 194-196)

Starkey 1999 (pp. 151-154)

Mastery and Demonstration

Practice and reinforce these competencies by reviewing your class notes and texts, observing peer teachers and certified/licensed professionals perform the skills, discussing the competencies with peer teachers and certified/licensed professionals, practicing alone and with a peer, and then demonstrating proficiency to a peer teacher. Finally, demonstrate your proficiency to an ACI.

Approved by (date and signature)

1. Background

    Peer _____

    ACI _____

2. Application

    Peer _____

    ACI _____

3. Maintenance

    Peer _____

    ACI _____

4. Recording

    Peer _____

    ACI _____

Comments

LEVEL 2

Module G4
Therapeutic Modalities

Cryotherapy

Objective

Develop and demonstrate the skills necessary to properly use cryotherapy during sport injury rehabilitation.

Competencies

1. Demonstrate and explain proper use of the following cryotherapy devices for treating an injury of your choice:

- Cold whirlpool treatment
- Controlled cold therapy unit
- Ice pack
- Vapo-coolant spray
- Ice immersion
- Ice massage

    a. Define the modality and briefly explain its effects, advantages, disadvantages, indications, contraindications, and precautions.

    b. Demonstrate preapplication procedures, including reevaluating the injury, evaluating results of previous treatment, setting and evaluating goals, selecting proper modality, and preparing the modality and patient.

    c. Demonstrate and explain proper application procedures, including turn on, adjustments, dosage, duration, and frequency of application.

    d. Demonstrate and explain proper postapplication procedures, including patient and equipment cleanup, instructions to the patient, and scheduling the next appointment.

    e. Demonstrate proper recording of these treatments on athletic training clinic forms.

References

Denegar 2000 (pp. 104-112)

Knight 1995 (pp. 43-58, 217-232)

Prentice 1999b (pp. 173-190)

Starkey 1999 (pp. 110-120, 129-142)

Mastery and Demonstration

Practice and reinforce these competencies by reviewing your class notes and texts, observing peer teachers and certified/licensed professionals perform the skills, discussing the competencies with peer teachers and certified/licensed professionals, practicing alone and with a peer, and then demonstrating proficiency to a peer teacher. Finally, demonstrate your proficiency to an ACI.

Approved by (date and signature)

1a-e. Complete competencies 1a-e for each of the following cryotherapy modalities.

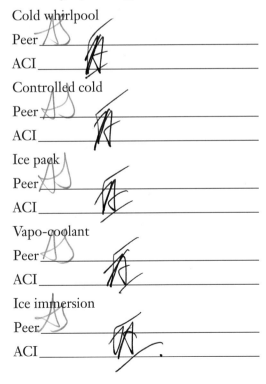

Cold whirlpool
Peer _____
ACI _____

Controlled cold
Peer _____
ACI _____

Ice pack
Peer _____
ACI _____

Vapo-coolant
Peer _____
ACI _____

Ice immersion
Peer _____
ACI _____

Ice massage

Peer _MG_

ACI _____

Comments

Cryokinetics

Objective

Develop and demonstrate the skills necessary to properly use cryokinetics during acute joint sprain rehabilitation.

Competencies

1. Define cryokinetics and briefly explain the following:

   a. Effects

   b. Advantages

   c. Disadvantages

   d. Indications

   e. Contraindications

   f. Precautions

2. Demonstrate and explain cryokinetic treatments for an ankle sprain and for a finger sprain. Include each of the following for each treatment:

   a. Preapplication procedures, including reevaluating the injury, evaluating results of previous treatment, setting and evaluating goals, selecting proper modality and temperature, and preparing the modality and patient.

   b. Application procedures, duration, and frequency of application.

   c. Postapplication procedures, including patient and equipment cleanup, instructions to the patient, and scheduling the next appointment.

3. Demonstrate proper recording of these treatments on athletic training clinic forms.

References

Denegar 2000 (pp. 110-111)

Knight 1995 (pp. 43-58, 217-232)

Prentice 1999b (pp. 189-190)

Mastery and Demonstration

Practice and reinforce these competencies by reviewing your class notes and texts, observing peer teachers and certified/licensed professionals perform the skills, discussing the competencies with peer teachers and certified/licensed professionals, practicing alone and with a peer, and then demonstrating proficiency to a peer teacher. Finally, demonstrate your proficiency to an ACI.

Approved by (date and signature)

1. Background

   Peer _____

   ACI _____

2a-b. Application

   Peer _____

   ACI _____

2c. Maintenance

   Peer _____

   ACI _____

3. Recording

   Peer _____

   ACI _____

Comments

LEVEL 2

Cryostretch

Objective

Develop and demonstrate the skills necessary to properly use cryostretch during acute muscle strain rehabilitation.

Competencies

1. Define cryostretch and briefly explain the following:

  a. Effects

  b. Advantages

  c. Disadvantages

  d. Indications

  e. Contraindications

  f. Precautions

2. Demonstrate and explain the following in relation to using cryostretch to treat a hamstring strain:

  a. Preapplication procedures, including re-evaluating the injury, evaluating results of previous treatment, setting and evaluating goals, selecting proper modality, and preparing the modality and patient.

  b. Application procedures, duration, and frequency of application.

  c. Postapplication procedures, including patient and equipment cleanup, instructions to the patient, and scheduling the next appointment.

3. For a hamstring strain and a triceps strain, demonstrate proper recording of these treatments on athletic training clinic forms.

References

Knight 1995 (pp. 43-58, 233-239)

Starkey 1999 (pp. 140-141)

Mastery and Demonstration

Practice and reinforce these competencies by reviewing your class notes and texts, observing peer teachers and certified/licensed professionals perform the skills, discussing the competencies with peer teachers and certified/licensed professionals, practicing alone and with a peer, and then demonstrating proficiency to a peer teacher. Finally, demonstrate your proficiency to an ACI.

Approved by (date and signature)

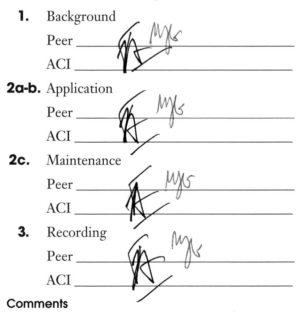

1. Background

  Peer _____

  ACI _____

2a-b. Application

  Peer _____

  ACI _____

2c. Maintenance

  Peer _____

  ACI _____

3. Recording

  Peer _____

  ACI _____

Comments

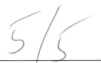

Intermittent Compression Devices

Objective

Develop and demonstrate the skills necessary to properly use an intermittent compression device during sport injury rehabilitation.

Competencies

1. Define intermittent compression devices and briefly explain the following:

    a. Therapeutic effects

    b. Advantages

    c. Disadvantages

    d. Indications

    e. Contraindications

    f. Precautions

2. Demonstrate and explain the following in relation to treating a hand contusion with an intermittent compression device:

    a. Preapplication procedures, including re-evaluating the injury, evaluating results of previous treatment, setting and evaluating goals, selecting proper modality, and preparing the modality and patient.

    b. Application procedures, including turn on, adjustments, dosage, duration, and frequency of application.

    c. Postapplication procedures, including patient and equipment cleanup, instructions to the patient, and scheduling the next appointment.

3. Demonstrate and explain maintenance and simple repair procedures for intermittent compression devices.

4. Demonstrate proper recording of intermittent compression device treatments on athletic training clinic forms.

References

Denegar 2000 (pp. 192-193)

Prentice 1999b (pp. 307-319)

Starkey 1999 (pp. 303-307)

Mastery and Demonstration

Practice and reinforce these competencies by reviewing your class notes and texts, observing peer teachers and certified/licensed professionals perform the skills, discussing the competencies with peer teachers and certified/licensed professionals, practicing alone and with a peer, and then demonstrating proficiency to a peer teacher. Finally, demonstrate your proficiency to an ACI.

Approved by (date and signature)

1. Background

    Peer _____

    ACI _____

2a-b. Application

    Peer _____

    ACI _____

2c-3. Maintenance

    Peer _____

    ACI _____

4. Recording

    Peer _____

    ACI _____

Comments

Ultrasound

Objective

Develop and demonstrate the skills necessary to properly use ultrasound during sport injury rehabilitation.

Competencies

1. Define and briefly explain the following:

   a. Thermal ultrasound treatment

   b. Nonthermal ultrasound treatment

   c. Combination electrical-stimulation/ultrasound treatment

   d. Phonophoresis treatment

   e. Indirect application of ultrasound treatment (underwater, bladder)

2. For each of the types of ultrasound in Competency 1, explain the following:

   a. Therapeutic effects

   b. Advantages

   c. Disadvantages

   d. Indications

   e. Contraindications

   f. Precautions

3. For each of the types of ultrasound in Competency 1, demonstrate and explain the following for treating injuries of your choice:

   a. Preapplication procedures, including re-evaluating the injury, evaluating results of previous treatment, setting/evaluating goals, selecting proper modality, and preparing the modality and patient.

   b. Application procedures, including turn on, adjustments, dosage, duration, and frequency of application.

   c. Postapplication procedures, including patient and equipment cleanup, instructions to the patient, and scheduling the next appointment.

4. Demonstrate and explain maintenance and simple repair procedures for ultrasound machines.

5. Demonstrate proper recording of ultrasound treatments on athletic training clinic forms.

References

Denegar 2000 (pp. 158-167)

Prentice 1999b (pp. 207-244)

Starkey 1999 (pp. 269-302)

Mastery and Demonstration

Practice and reinforce these competencies by reviewing your class notes and texts, observing peer teachers and certified/licensed professionals perform the skills, discussing the competencies with peer teachers and certified/licensed professionals, practicing alone and with a peer, and then demonstrating proficiency to a peer teacher. Finally, demonstrate your proficiency to an ACI.

Approved by (date and signature)

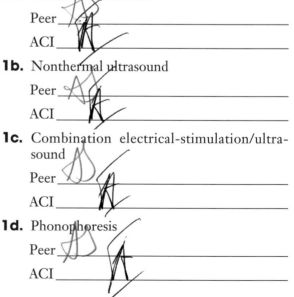

1a. Thermal ultrasound

Peer _____

ACI _____

1b. Nonthermal ultrasound

Peer _____

ACI _____

1c. Combination electrical-stimulation/ultrasound

Peer _____

ACI _____

1d. Phonophoresis

Peer _____

ACI _____

1e. Indirect application

Peer _____

ACI _____

Comments

Diathermy

Objective

Develop and demonstrate the skills necessary to properly use diathermy during sport injury rehabilitation.

Competencies

1. Define and briefly explain the following:

   a. Microwave diathermy

   b. Pulsed short-wave diathermy

2. For each of the two types of diathermy in Competency 1, explain the following:

   a. Therapeutic effects

   b. Advantages

   c. Disadvantages

   d. Indications

   e. Contraindications

   f. Precautions

3. For each of the two types of diathermy in Competency 1, demonstrate and explain the following for treating injuries of your choice:

   a. Preapplication procedures, including re-evaluating the injury, evaluating results of previous treatment, setting and evaluating goals, selecting proper modality, and preparing the modality and patient.

   b. Application procedures, including turn on, adjustments, dosage, duration, and frequency of application.

   c. Postapplication procedures, including patient and equipment cleanup, instructions to the patient, and scheduling the next appointment.

4. Demonstrate and explain maintenance and simple repair procedures for diathermy machines.

5. Demonstrate proper recording of diathermy treatments on athletic training clinic forms.

References

Denegar 2000 (pp. 168-172)

Prentice 1999b (pp. 148-167)

Starkey 1999 (pp. 155-163)

Mastery and Demonstration

Practice and reinforce these competencies by reviewing your class notes and texts, observing peer teachers and certified/licensed professionals perform the skills, discussing the competencies with peer teachers and certified/licensed professionals, practicing alone and with a peer, and then demonstrating proficiency to a peer teacher. Finally, demonstrate your proficiency to an ACI.

Approved by (date and signature)

1-2. Background

   Peer _____

   ACI _____

3. Application

   Peer _____

   ACI _____

4. Maintenance

   Peer _____

   ACI _____

5. Recording

   Peer _____

   ACI _____

Comments

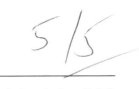

LEVEL 2

Module G10
Therapeutic Modalities

Electrical Stimulation

Objective

Develop and demonstrate the skills necessary to properly use electrical stimulation during sport injury rehabilitation.

Competencies

1. Define and briefly explain the use of electrical stimulation, including the type of electrical stimulator and its specific settings, you would use to achieve the following:

   a. Sensory-level pain control

   b. Noxious-level pain control

   c. Motor-level pain control

   d. Muscle reeducation

   e. Muscle pumping

   f. Muscle atrophy retardation

   g. Acute edema reduction

   h. Muscle splinting/spasm reduction

   i. Iontophoresis

2. For each of the goals of electrical stimulation in Competency 1, demonstrate and explain the following, using the proper electrical simulator to treat injuries of your choice:

   - Preapplication procedures, including reevaluating the injury, evaluating results of previous treatment, setting and evaluating goals, selecting proper modality, and preparing the modality and patient.

   - Application procedures, including turn on, adjustments, dosage, duration, and frequency of application.

   - Postapplication procedures, including patient and equipment cleanup, instructions to the patient, and scheduling the next appointment.

   - Maintenance and simple repair procedures for electrical muscle stimulation machines.

   - Proper recording of electrical stimulation treatments on athletic training clinic forms.

3. For each of the following electrical stimulation units not used in Competency 2, demonstrate and explain its proper use to achieve one of the goals in Competency 1.

   a. Monophasic stimulator (e.g., high-volt stimulation)

   b. Biphasic stimulator (e.g., transcutaneous electrical nerve stimulation [TENS] and neuromuscular electrical stimulation [NMES])

   c. Direct current (e.g., iontophoresis)

   d. Alternating current (e.g., interferential, NMES)

   e. Multifunction electrical stimulation devices

References

Denegar 2000 (pp. 126-155)

Prentice 1999b (pp. 52-125)

Starkey 1999 (pp. 170-258)

Mastery and Demonstration

Practice and reinforce these competencies by reviewing your class notes and texts, observing peer teachers and certified/licensed professionals perform the skills, discussing the competencies with peer teachers and certified/licensed professionals, practicing alone and with a peer, and then demonstrating proficiency to a peer teacher. Finally, demonstrate your proficiency to an ACI.

Approved by (date and signature)

1-2. Complete competencies 1 and 2 for each of the following:

   a. Sensory-level pain control

   Peer _____

   ACI _____

83

b. Noxious-level pain control

Peer _____

ACI _____

c. Motor-level pain control

Peer _____

ACI _____

d. Muscle reeducation

Peer _____

ACI _____

e. Muscle pumping

Peer _____

ACI _____

f. Muscle atrophy retardation

Peer _____

ACI _____

g. Acute edema reduction

Peer _____

ACI _____

h. Muscle splinting/spasm reduction

Peer _____

ACI _____

i. Iontophoresis

Peer _____

ACI _____

3a. Monophasic stimulator

Peer _____

ACI _____

3b. Biphasic stimulator

Peer _____

ACI _____

3c. Direct current

Peer _____

ACI _____

3d. Alternating current

Peer _____

ACI _____

3e. Multifunction electrical stimulation devices

Peer _____

ACI _____

Comments

Therapeutic Massage

Objective

Develop and demonstrate the skills necessary to properly use massage during sport injury rehabilitation.

Competencies

1. Define, briefly explain, and differentiate between the following massage strokes:

   a. Effleurage

   b. Petrissage

   c. Friction (circular, transverse) - tendon *good for*   *rest if stretched*

   d. Tapotement - rehab

   e. Vibration

   f. Myofascial release techniques - release muscle tension due to Fascia

2. For each of the massage strokes in Competency 1, explain the following:

   • Therapeutic effects

   • Advantages

   • Disadvantages

   • Indications

   • Contraindications

   • Precautions

3. Demonstrate each of the massage strokes in Competency 1.

4. Demonstrate and explain an overall or integrated therapeutic massage treatment including the following:

   a. Preapplication procedures, including re-evaluating the injury, evaluating results of previous treatment, setting and evaluating goals, selecting proper modality, and preparing patient.

   b. Application procedures, including types and sequence of strokes, adjustments, duration, and frequency of application.

   c. Postapplication procedures, including patient and equipment cleanup, instructions

to the patient, and scheduling the next appointment.

   d. Proper recording of massage treatments on athletic training clinic forms.

References

Denegar 2000 (pp. 177-184)

Houglum 2001 (pp. 155-158)

Prentice 1999b (pp. 320-341)

Starkey 1999 (pp. 329-339)

Mastery and Demonstration

Practice and reinforce these competencies by reviewing your class notes and texts, observing peer teachers and certified/licensed professionals perform the skills, discussing the competencies with peer teachers and certified/licensed professionals, practicing alone and with a peer, and then demonstrating proficiency to a peer teacher. Finally, demonstrate your proficiency to an ACI.

Approved by (date and signature)

1-3. Complete competencies 1 through 3 for each of the following massage strokes:

   a. Effleurage

   Peer_____

   ACI_____

   b. Petrissage

   Peer_____

   ACI_____

   c. Friction (circular, transverse)

   Peer_____

   ACI_____

   d. Tapotement

   Peer_____

   ACI_____

e. Vibration

Peer _____

ACI _____

f. Myofascial release techniques

Peer _____

ACI _____

4. Overall massage

Peer _____

ACI _____

Comments

Traction

Objective

Develop and demonstrate the skills necessary to properly use traction during sport injury rehabilitation.

Competencies

1. Define, briefly explain, and differentiate between the following:

a. Mechanical traction

b. Manual traction

c. Positional traction

2. For each of the three types of traction in Competency 1, explain the following:

- Therapeutic effects

- Advantages

- Disadvantages

- Indications

- Contraindications

- Precautions

3. For each of the three types of traction in Competency 1, demonstrate and explain the following:

- Preapplication procedures, including reevaluating the injury, evaluating results of previous treatment, setting and evaluating goals, selecting proper modality, and preparing the modality and patient.

- Application procedures, including turn on, adjustments, dosage, duration, and frequency of application.

- Postapplication procedures, including patient and equipment cleanup, instructions to the patient, and scheduling the next appointment.

4. Demonstrate and explain maintenance and simple repair procedures for traction devices.

5. Demonstrate proper recording of traction treatments on athletic training clinic forms.

References

Denegar 2000 (pp. 184-192)

Prentice 1999b (pp. 284-306)

Starkey 1999 (pp. 326-328)

Mastery and Demonstration

Practice and reinforce these competencies by reviewing your class notes and texts, observing peer teachers and certified/licensed professionals perform the skills, discussing the competencies with peer teachers and certified/licensed professionals, practicing alone and with a peer, and then demonstrating proficiency to a peer teacher. Finally, demonstrate your proficiency to an ACI.

Approved by (date and signature)

1-3. Complete competencies 1 through 3 for each of the following types of traction:

a. Mechanical traction

Peer _____

ACI _____

b. Manual traction

Peer _____

ACI _____

c. Positional traction

Peer _____

ACI _____

4. Maintenance

Peer _____

ACI _____

5. Recording

    Peer _____

    ACI _____

Comments

Rehabilitation Overview

Objective

Demonstrate the ability to design an overall rehabilitation program that will progress an athlete from injury to full sport participation.

Competencies

1. Outline an overall rehabilitation program for an injury of your choice. Include the following components:

   a. Phases or elements

   b. Goal of each phase

   c. Specific tools you would use for each phase (e.g., therapeutic modalities, therapeutic exercise)

   d. Criteria for progressing from phase to phase

   e. Assessment tools you would use to determine if your patient had met the progression criteria

2. Discuss the roles of other professionals (e.g., physicians, physical therapists, exercise physiologists) in athletic and sport rehabilitation.

References

Denegar 2000 (pp. 12-27)

Houglum 2001 (pp. 2-29, 61-62)

Knight 1995 (pp. 43-57)

Prentice 1999a (pp. 2-39)

Mastery and Demonstration

Practice and reinforce these competencies by reviewing your class notes and texts, observing peer teachers and certified/licensed professionals perform the skills, discussing the competencies with peer teachers and certified/licensed professionals, practicing alone and with a peer, and then demonstrating proficiency to a peer teacher. Finally, demonstrate your proficiency to an ACI.

Approved by (date and signature)

1. Overall plan

   Peer _____

   ACI _____

2. Other professionals

   Peer _____

   ACI _____

Comments

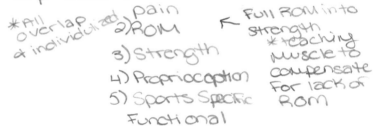

a. phases -1) inflammation
*All overlap + individualized 2) pain 2) ROM ← Full ROM into strength *teaching muscle to compensate for lack of ROM
3) Strength
4) Proprioception
5) Sports Specific Functional

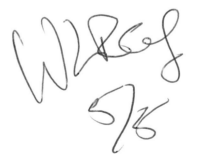

1/18/11

Rehabilitation Adherence and Motivation Techniques

Objective

Demonstrate the ability to motivate an athlete during a rehabilitation session.

Competencies

1. Demonstrate use of the following motivational techniques during rehabilitation:
   a. Verbal motivation
   b. Visualization
   c. Imagery
   d. Desensitization *- get them through DABDA*

2. Discuss techniques of increasing patient compliance with rehabilitation.

References

Denegar 2000 (pp. 12-27)

Houglum 2001 (pp. 55-63)

Prentice 1999a (pp. 40-60)

Mastery and Demonstration

Practice and reinforce these competencies by reviewing your class notes and texts, observing peer teachers and certified/licensed professionals perform the skills, discussing the competencies with peer teachers and certified/licensed professionals, practicing alone and with a peer, and then demonstrating proficiency to a peer teacher. Finally, demonstrate your proficiency to an ACI.

Approved by (date and signature)

1a. Verbal motivation

Peer _____

ACI _____

1b. Visualization

Peer _____

ACI _____

1c. Imagery

Peer _____

ACI _____

1d. Desensitization

Peer _____

ACI _____

2. Patient compliance

Peer _____

ACI _____

Comments

*DABDA
Denial
A
Bargining
Depression
Acceptance*

*WL&Cf
5/5*

PROM
&
AROM &Shoulder -list them
make copies
-outline
1/18/11

LEVEL 2   Module H3
Therapeutic Exercise

Range of Motion and Flexibility Exercises

Objective

Develop and demonstrate the skills necessary to properly use therapeutic exercise to improve ROM and flexibility during sport injury rehabilitation.

Competencies

1. Discuss the role of improving ROM and flexibility during sport injury rehabilitation, including when during the rehabilitation process it should be performed.

2. Discuss the difference between anatomic and functional ROM and give examples of each.

3. Discuss the role of joint mobilization in increasing ROM and flexibility.

4. Demonstrate proper use of a goniometer to measure ROM at three different joints.

5. Demonstrate proper use of each of the following types of therapeutic exercise for improving upper extremity ROM and flexibility:

   a. Passive ROM

   b. Active ROM

   c. Active-assisted ROM

   by performing each of the elements of therapeutic exercise in this list:

   - Position the patient.
   - Stabilize the patient during repetitions.
   - Demonstrate and instruct proper execution of repetitions (form, timing, control).
   - Explain how and when to adjust the exercise.
   - Demonstrate ways an athlete can "cheat" while performing the exercise.
   - Outline safety factors for the athlete and yourself.
   - Demonstrate how to record results of this type of therapeutic exercise session.

6. Demonstrate proper use of each of the following types of therapeutic exercise for improving lower extremity ROM and flexibility:

   a. Passive ROM

   b. Active ROM

   c. Active-assisted ROM

   by performing each of the elements of therapeutic exercise in the list in Competency 5.

7. Demonstrate proper use of each of the following types of therapeutic exercise for improving trunk extremity ROM and flexibility:

   a. Passive ROM

   b. Active ROM

   c. Active-assisted ROM

   by performing each of the elements of therapeutic exercise in the list in Competency 5.

8. Demonstrate proper use of each of the following types of therapeutic exercise for improving cervical spine ROM and flexibility:

   a. Passive ROM

   b. Active ROM

   c. Active-assisted ROM

   by performing each of the elements of therapeutic exercise in the list in Competency 5.

References

Allsen, Harrison, and Vance 1997 (pp. 190-215)

Arnheim and Prentice 2000 (pp. 76-87)

Houglum 2001 (pp. 120-150)

Prentice 1999a (pp. 62-72)

Mastery and Demonstration

Practice and reinforce these competencies by reviewing your class notes and texts, observing peer teachers and certified/licensed professionals perform the skills, discussing the competencies with peer teachers and certified/licensed professionals, practicing alone and with a peer, and then demonstrating proficiency to a peer teacher. Finally, demonstrate your proficiency to an ACI.

Approved by (date and signature)

1. Background

Peer _____

ACI _____

2. Anatomic vs. physiologic

Peer _____

ACI _____

3. Role of joint mobilization

Peer _____

ACI _____

4. Goniometer

Peer _____

ACI _____

5a. Upper extremity—passive ROM

Peer _____

ACI _____

5b. Upper extremity—active ROM

Peer _____

ACI _____

5c. Upper extremity—active-assisted ROM

Peer _____

ACI _____

6a. Lower extremity—passive ROM

Peer _____

ACI _____

6b. Lower extremity—active ROM

Peer _____

ACI _____

6c. Lower extremity—active-assisted ROM

Peer _____

ACI _____

7a. Trunk—passive ROM

Peer _____

ACI _____

7b. Trunk—active ROM

Peer _____

ACI _____

7c. Trunk—active-assisted ROM

Peer _____

ACI _____

8a. Cervical spine—passive ROM

Peer _____

ACI _____

8b. Cervical spine—active ROM

Peer _____

ACI _____

8c. Cervical spine—active-assisted ROM

Peer _____

ACI _____

Comments

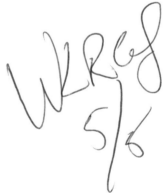

Athletic Apparel nextweek

Therapeutic Exercise

Joint Mobilization

surgery not advised due stress on repaired structures

Objective

Develop and demonstrate the skills necessary to properly use mobilization during sport injury rehabilitation.

Competencies

1. Define and briefly explain mobilization, including the following:

   a. Therapeutic effects

   b. Advantages

   c. Disadvantages

   d. Indications

   e. Contraindications

   f. Precautions

   - Takes awhile
   - Trainer dependent
   - Advanced tech
   - Clinic'l are not great candidates

2. Define and demonstrate:

   a. Loose and close packed positions

   b. Joint play

   c. Roll, glide, spin

   d. Concave and convex rules

   e. Long-axis distraction

   f. Glides (e.g., anterior/posterior, superior/inferior)

   c packed
   ax amount
   nt space
   scles loose
   ed packed
   uscles are
   ight

3. Define and demonstrate grades I-IV of mobilization as defined by Maitland by doing each of the following:

   • Preapplication procedures, including reevaluating the injury, evaluating results of previous treatment, setting and evaluating goals, selecting proper modality, and preparing the patient.

   • Application procedures, hand placement, force, repetitions, adjustments, duration, and frequency of application.

   • Postapplication procedures, including patient cleanup, instructions to the patient, and scheduling the next appointment.

   • Proper recording of joint mobilization treatments on athletic training clinic forms.

4. Define and demonstrate self-mobilization for a body part of your choice.

References

Arnheim and Prentice 2000 (pp. 397-400)

Houglum 2001 (pp. 154-200)

Prentice 1999a (pp. 188-197)

Grade 1+2
- stimulating pn receptors
- moves fluid around

Mastery and Demonstration

Practice and reinforce these competencies by reviewing your class notes and texts, observing peer teachers and certified/licensed professionals perform the skills, discussing the competencies with peer teachers and certified/licensed professionals, practicing alone and with a peer, and then demonstrating proficiency to a peer teacher. Finally, demonstrate your proficiency to an ACI.

Approved by (date and signature)

1. Background

   Peer_____

   ACI_____

2a. Loose and close-packed positions

   Peer_____

   ACI_____

2b. Joint play

   Peer_____

   ACI_____

2c. Roll, glide, spin

   Peer_____

   ACI_____

2d. Concave and convex rules

   Peer_____

   ACI_____

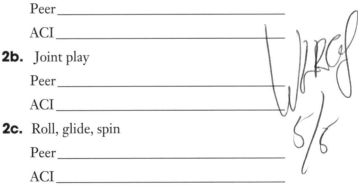

concave *convex*

Roll- Shoulder Abd/Add
Knee - Squat
Slide- Knee- leg extension
Ankle- moving into DF seated
Spin- Shoulder Flex/Ext
Glide- Ankle → Squat

2e. Long-axis distraction

Peer _____

ACI _____

2f. Glides (e.g., anterior/posterior, superior/in-ferior)

Peer _____

ACI _____

3. Maitland—grade I

Peer _____

ACI _____

Maitland—grade II

Peer _____

ACI _____

Maitland—grade III

Peer _____

ACI _____

Maitland—grade IV

Peer _____

ACI _____

4. Self-mobilization

Peer _____

ACI _____

Comments

Isometric Resistance Exercises

Objective

Develop and demonstrate the skills necessary to properly use isometric resistance exercises during sport injury rehabilitation.

Competencies

1. Discuss isometric resistance, how it is developed, the equipment needed, and its similarities to and differences from isotonic and isokinetic resistance.

2. Demonstrate proper use of isometrics for strengthening the following:

   a. Lower extremity

   b. Upper extremity

   c. Cervical spine

   d. Trunk and torso

   by doing each of the following for each exercise:

   - Set up the equipment.
   - Position the patient.
   - Stabilize the patient during repetitions.
   - Demonstrate and instruct proper execution of repetitions (form, timing, control).
   - Explain how and when to adjust the equipment.
   - Demonstrate ways an athlete can cheat on the equipment.
   - Outline safety factors for the athlete and yourself.
   - Demonstrate how to record results of this type of therapeutic exercise session.
   - Demonstrate and explain maintenance and simple repair procedures for the equipment.

References

Houglum 2001 (pp. 202-264)

Kisner and Colby 1996 (pp. 72-83)

Prentice 1999a (pp. 73-78, 314-322, 513-516)

Mastery and Demonstration

Practice and reinforce these competencies by reviewing your class notes and texts, observing peer teachers and certified/licensed professionals perform the skills, discussing the competencies with peer teachers and certified/licensed professionals, practicing alone and with a peer, and then demonstrating proficiency to a peer teacher. Finally, demonstrate your proficiency to an ACI.

Approved by (date and signature)

1. Background

   Peer _____

   ACI _____

2a. Application—lower extremity

   Peer _____

   ACI _____

2b. Application—upper extremity

   Peer _____

   ACI _____

2c. Application—cervical spine

   Peer _____

   ACI _____

2d. Application—trunk and torso

   Peer _____

   ACI _____

Comments

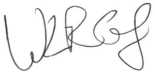

Therapeutic Exercise

Isotonic Strength-Training Devices

Objective

Develop and demonstrate the skills necessary to properly use isotonic devices to develop strength during sport injury rehabilitation.

Competencies

1. Discuss isotonic resistance, how it is developed, the equipment needed, and its similarities to and differences from isometric and isokinetic resistance.

2. Demonstrate proper use of isotonic weight training equipment for strengthening the following:

   a. Knee and thigh (using a knee flexion and extension machine)

   b. Overall legs (leg press or squat)

   c. Shoulder (abduction, internal and external rotation)

   d. Trunk and torso

   e. Cervical spine

   by doing each of the following:

   - Set up the equipment.
   - Position the patient.
   - Stabilize the patient during repetitions.
   - Demonstrate proper execution of repetitions (form, timing, control).
   - Explain how and when to adjust the equipment.
   - Demonstrate ways an athlete can cheat on the equipment.
   - Outline safety factors for the athlete and yourself.
   - Demonstrate how to record results.
   - Demonstrate and explain maintenance and simple repair procedures.

References

Houglum 2001 (pp. 202-264)

Prentice 1999a (pp. 73-78, 314, 361, 412, 448, 491)

Mastery and Demonstration

Practice and reinforce these competencies by reviewing your class notes and texts, observing peer teachers and certified/licensed professionals perform the skills, discussing the competencies with peer teachers and certified/licensed professionals, practicing alone and with a peer, and then demonstrating proficiency to a peer teacher. Finally, demonstrate your proficiency to an ACI.

Approved by (date and signature)

1. Background

   Peer _____

   ACI _____

2a. Knee and thigh (using a knee flexion and extension machine)

   Peer _____

   ACI _____

2b. Overall legs (leg press or squat)

   Peer _____

   ACI _____

2c. Shoulder (abduction, internal and external rotation)

   Peer _____

   ACI _____

2d. Trunk and torso

   Peer _____

   ACI _____

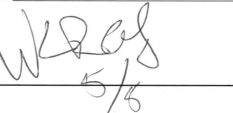

2e. Cervical spine

Peer _____

ACI _____

Comments

Daily Adjustable Progressive Exercise

Objective

Develop and demonstrate the skills necessary to properly use the daily adjustable progressive exercise (DAPRE) technique for evaluating and redeveloping strength during sport injury rehabilitation.

Competencies

1. Define the DAPRE technique and briefly explain the following:
    a. Effects
    b. Advantages
    c. Disadvantages
    d. Indications
    e. Contraindications
    f. Precautions

2. Explain why the DAPRE technique can only be used with isotonic and isometric equipment.

3. Explain the role of verbal encouragement during DAPRE and demonstrate how you verbally encourage an athlete to perform to his or her fullest.

4. Demonstrate and explain use of the DAPRE technique for the following:
    a. Knee strength development
    b. Ankle strength development
    c. Shoulder strength development

5. Demonstrate and explain how to use the DAPRE technique for strength maintenance.

6. Demonstrate and explain how to use the DAPRE technique to evaluate strength maintenance.

7. Demonstrate proper recording of these treatments on athletic training clinic forms.

References

Anderson, Hall, and Martin 2000 (pp. 170-171)

Knight 1995 (pp. 43-51)

Prentice 1999a (pp. 81-82)

Mastery and Demonstration

Practice and reinforce these competencies by reviewing your class notes and texts, observing peer teachers and certified/licensed professionals perform the skills, discussing the competencies with peer teachers and certified/licensed professionals, practicing alone and with a peer, and then demonstrating proficiency to a peer teacher. Finally, demonstrate your proficiency to an ACI.

Approved by (date and signature)

1. Background

    Peer_____

    ACI_____

2. Equipment

    Peer_____

    ACI_____

3. Verbal encouragement

    Peer_____

    ACI_____

4a. Knee application

    Peer_____

    ACI_____

4b. Ankle application

    Peer_____

    ACI_____

4c. Shoulder application

    Peer_____

    ACI_____

5. Maintenance

Peer_____

ACI_____

6. Evaluation

Peer_____

ACI_____

7. Recording

Peer_____

ACI_____

Comments

Isokinetic Dynamometers

Objective

Develop and demonstrate the skills necessary to properly use an isokinetic dynamometer to evaluate and develop strength during sport injury rehabilitation.

Competencies

1. Explain the similarities and differences between isotonic, isometric, and isokinetic resistance.

2. Discuss the similarities and differences between the three principle types of isokinetic dynamometers:

   a. Mechanical

   b. Electrical

   c. Computer generated

3. Demonstrate proper use of an isokinetic dynamometer for the following:

   a. Evaluating or measuring knee strength

   b. Evaluating or measuring shoulder strength

   c. Developing or training muscular strength by doing each of the following:

   - Set up the equipment.
   - Position the patient.
   - Stabilize the patient during repetitions.
   - Demonstrate proper execution of repetitions (form, timing, control).
   - Explain how and when to adjust the equipment.
   - Demonstrate ways an athlete can cheat on the equipment.
   - Outline safety factors for the athlete and yourself.
   - Demonstrate how to record results.
   - Demonstrate and explain maintenance and simple repair procedures.

References

Houglum 2001 (pp. 219-227, 248-250, 628, 685, 738, 874)

Perrin 1993 (pp. 1-69)

Prentice 1999a (pp. 146-156)

Mastery and Demonstration

Practice and reinforce these competencies by reviewing your class notes and texts, observing peer teachers and certified/licensed professionals perform the skills, discussing the competencies with peer teachers and certified/licensed professionals, practicing alone and with a peer, and then demonstrating proficiency to a peer teacher. Finally, demonstrate your proficiency to an ACI.

Approved by (date and signature)

1. Resistance types

   Peer _____

   ACI _____

2. Isokinetic devices

   Peer _____

   ACI _____

3a. Measure knee strength

   Peer _____

   ACI _____

3b. Measure shoulder strength

   Peer _____

   ACI _____

3c. Develop muscle strength

   Peer _____

   ACI _____

Comments

Muscular Endurance

Objective

Develop and demonstrate the skills necessary to properly use therapeutic exercise to improve muscular endurance during sport injury rehabilitation.

Competencies

1. Discuss the role of improving muscular endurance during sport injury rehabilitation, including when during the rehabilitation process such exercises should be performed.

2. Demonstrate proper use of the following therapeutic exercises for improving muscular endurance:

   a. Upper body
   - Aquatics
   - UBE/stationary bicycle
   - Physioballs

   b. Lower body
   - Aquatics
   - Stationary bicycle
   - Stair stepper
   - Physioballs

   by doing each of the following for each exercise:

   a. Set up the equipment.

   b. Position the patient.

   c. Stabilize the patient during repetitions.

   d. Demonstrate and instruct proper execution of repetitions (form, timing, control).

   e. Explain how and when to adjust the equipment.

   f. Demonstrate ways an athlete can cheat on the equipment.

   g. Outline safety factors for the athlete and yourself.

   h. Demonstrate how to record results of this type of therapeutic exercise session.

   i. Demonstrate and explain maintenance and simple repair procedures for the equipment.

References

Houglum 2001 (pp. 202-267, 442-473)

Prentice 1999a (pp. 73-86, 367)

Mastery and Demonstration

Practice and reinforce these competencies by reviewing your class notes and texts, observing peer teachers and certified/licensed professionals perform the skills, discussing the competencies with peer teachers and certified/licensed professionals, practicing alone and with a peer, and then demonstrating proficiency to a peer teacher. Finally, demonstrate your proficiency to an ACI.

Approved by (date and signature)

1. Background

   Peer _____

   ACI _____

2a. Upper body—aquatics

   Peer _____

   ACI _____

   Upper body—UBE/bike

   Peer _____

   ACI _____

   Upper body—physioballs

   Peer _____

   ACI _____

2b. Lower body—aquatics

   Peer _____

   ACI _____

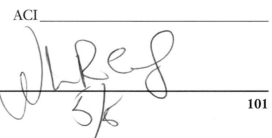

Lower body—bike

Peer _____

ACI _____

Lower body—stair stepper

Peer _____

ACI _____

Lower body—physioballs

Peer _____

ACI _____

Comments

WLRay

Aquatic Therapy

Objective

Develop and demonstrate the skills necessary to properly use pool therapy during sports injury rehabilitation.

Competencies

1. Define pool therapy and briefly explain the following:

   a. Effects

   b. Advantages

   c. Disadvantages

   d. Indications

   e. Contraindications

   f. Precautions

2. Demonstrate and explain the use of a swimming pool for the following:

   a. Increasing joint ROM

   b. Developing muscular endurance

   c. Developing cardiovascular endurance

   d. Relieving general muscular soreness

   e. Relieving general mental fatigue

3. For each condition, demonstrate and explain the following:

   a. Preapplication procedures

   b. Application procedures

   c. Postapplication procedures

4. Demonstrate proper recording of these treatments on athletic training clinic forms.

References

Arnheim and Prentice 2000 (pp. 392-394)

Houglum 2001 (pp. 406-441)

Prentice 1999a (pp. 217-225)

Mastery and Demonstration

Practice and reinforce these competencies by reviewing your class notes and texts, observing peer teachers and certified/licensed professionals perform the skills, discussing the competencies with peer teachers and certified/licensed professionals, practicing alone and with a peer, and then demonstrating proficiency to a peer teacher. Finally, demonstrate your proficiency to an ACI.

Approved by (date and signature)

1. Background

   Peer _____

   ACI _____

2a. Increase ROM

   Peer _____

   ACI _____

2b. Develop muscular endurance

   Peer _____

   ACI _____

2c. Develop cardiovascular endurance

   Peer _____

   ACI _____

2d. Relieve general muscle soreness

   Peer _____

   ACI _____

2e. Relieve mental fatigue

   Peer _____

   ACI _____

3. Application

   Peer _____

   ACI _____

4. Recording   **Comments**

Peer _____

ACI _____ _WRG_ _____

Neuromuscular Control and Coordination Exercises

Objective

Develop and demonstrate the skills necessary to properly use therapeutic exercise to improve neuromuscular control and coordination during sport injury rehabilitation.

Competencies

1. Discuss the role of improving neuromuscular control and coordination during sport injury rehabilitation, including when during the rehabilitation process it should be performed.

2. Demonstrate proper use of the following therapeutic exercises for improving neuromuscular control and coordination:

   a. Upper body
   - Proprioceptive neuromuscular facilitation (PNF) patterns
   - Proprioception board or balance
   - Double- and single-arm balancing
   - Wobble board or balance apparatus
   - Weighted-ball rebounding or toss

   b. Lower body
   - PNF patterns
   - Rhythmic stabilization apparatus
   - Incline board
   - Single-leg balancing

   c. Neck
   - Stabilization
   - Postural correction

   d. Trunk
   - Stabilization
   - Postural correction

   by doing each of the following for each exercise:

   - Set up the equipment, if necessary.

   - Position the patient.
   - Stabilize the patient during repetitions.
   - Demonstrate and instruct proper execution of repetitions (form, timing, control).
   - Explain how and when to adjust the exercise.
   - Demonstrate ways an athlete can cheat while performing the exercise.
   - Outline safety factors for the athlete and yourself.
   - Demonstrate how to record results of this type of therapeutic exercise session.
   - Demonstrate and explain maintenance and simple repair procedures for the equipment.

References

Houglum 2001 (pp. 266-283)

Perrin 1995 (pp. 1-69)

Prentice 1999a (pp. 82-132)

Mastery and Demonstration

Practice and reinforce these competencies by reviewing your class notes and texts, observing peer teachers and certified/licensed professionals perform the skills, discussing the competencies with peer teachers and certified/licensed professionals, practicing alone and with a peer, and then demonstrating proficiency to a peer teacher. Finally, demonstrate your proficiency to an ACI.

Approved by (date and signature)

1. Background

   Peer _____

   ACI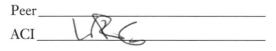

2a. Upper body—PNF patterns

Peer _____

ACI _____ WRG _____

Upper body—proprioception

Peer _____

ACI _____ WRG _____

Upper body—arm balance

Peer _____

ACI _____ WRG _____

Upper body—balance apparatus

Peer _____

ACI _____ WRG _____

Upper body—weighted ball toss

Peer _____

ACI _____ WRG _____

2b. Lower body—PNF patterns

Peer _____

ACI _____ WRG _____

Lower body—rhythmic stabilization

Peer _____

ACI _____ WRG _____

Lower body—incline board

Peer _____

ACI _____ WRG _____

Lower body—single-leg balance

Peer _____

ACI _____ WRG _____

2c. Neck stabilization

Peer _____

ACI _____ WRG _____

Neck postural correction

Peer _____

ACI _____ WRG _____

2d. Trunk stabilization

Peer _____

ACI _____ WRG _____

Trunk postural correction

Peer _____

ACI _____ WRG _____

Comments

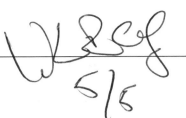

W?eg
5/5

Muscular Speed Exercises

Objective

Develop and demonstrate the skills necessary to properly use therapeutic exercise to improve muscular speed during sport injury rehabilitation.

Competencies

1. Discuss the role of improving muscular speed during sport injury rehabilitation, including when during the rehabilitation process it should be performed.

2. Demonstrate proper use of the following therapeutic exercises for improving muscular speed:

   a. Reaction drills—upper body

   b. Reaction drills—lower body

   c. Sprint work

   d. Fartlek training

   by doing each of the following for each exercise:

   • Set up the equipment.

   • Position the patient.

   • Stabilize the patient during repetitions.

   • Demonstrate and instruct proper execution of repetitions (form, timing, control).

   • Explain how and when to adjust the equipment.

   • Demonstrate ways an athlete can cheat on the equipment.

   • Outline safety factors for the athlete and yourself.

   • Demonstrate how to record results of this type of therapeutic exercise session.

   • Demonstrate and explain maintenance and simple repair procedures for the equipment.

References

Houglum 2001 (pp. 218, 277, 321)

Mastery and Demonstration

Practice and reinforce these competencies by reviewing your class notes and texts, observing peer teachers and certified/licensed professionals perform the skills, discussing the competencies with peer teachers and certified/licensed professionals, practicing alone and with a peer, and then demonstrating proficiency to a peer teacher. Finally, demonstrate your proficiency to an ACI.

Approved by (date and signature)

1. Background

   Peer _____

   ACI _____

2a. Reaction—upper body

   Peer _____

   ACI _____

2b. Reaction—lower body

   Peer _____

   ACI _____

2c. Sprint

   Peer _____

   ACI _____

2d. Fartlek

   Peer _____

   ACI _____

Comments

Train muscle to fire as fast as possible
-combining plyos & agility
Reaction drills-*hand eye coordination
  -Dot drill
  - boxes

D. Fartlek training
  -short increases in activity over a long peroid
    of time
  -Indian Run (example)
  -trains muscles to work harder when tired

  - Stadium Run (example)

*change of direction (measured in time)
* not looking at loading like plyos

Agility Exercises

Objective

Develop and demonstrate the skills necessary to properly use therapeutic exercise to improve agility during sport injury rehabilitation.

Competencies

1. Discuss the role of improving agility during sport injury rehabilitation, including when during the rehabilitation process it should be performed.

2. Demonstrate proper use of the following therapeutic exercises for improving agility:

a. Upper body

- Throwing
- Catching

b. Lower body

- Carioca
- Crossover
- Figure eight

by doing each of the following for each exercise:

- Set up the equipment, if necessary.
- Position the patient.
- Stabilize the patient during repetitions.
- Demonstrate and instruct proper execution of repetitions (form, timing, control).
- Explain how and when to adjust the exercise.
- Demonstrate ways an athlete can cheat while performing the exercise.
- Outline safety factors for the athlete and yourself.
- Demonstrate how to record results of this type of therapeutic exercise session.
- Demonstrate and explain maintenance and simple repair procedures for the equipment.

References

Houglum 2001 (pp. 277, 319-328, 805-809, 875)

Prentice 1999a (pp. 279-280)

Mastery and Demonstration

Practice and reinforce these competencies by reviewing your class notes and texts, observing peer teachers and certified/licensed professionals perform the skills, discussing the competencies with peer teachers and certified/licensed professionals, practicing alone and with a peer, and then demonstrating proficiency to a peer teacher. Finally, demonstrate your proficiency to an ACI.

Approved by (date and signature)

1. Background

Peer _____

ACI _____

2a. Upper body—throwing

Peer _____

ACI _____

Upper body—catching

Peer _____

ACI _____

2b. Lower body—carioca

Peer _____

ACI _____

Lower body—crossover

Peer _____

ACI _____

Lower body—figure eight

Peer _____

ACI _____

Comments

phase
Ammorization - switching from eccentric to concentric
- theory - more eccentric load the greater the power w/ a shorter ammorization phase

 Jumping down from box & jumping right away (eccentric) (how fast load to conc)

Plyometrics

Sport-Fitness-advisor.com/plyometric-drills.html

...ons.

3. Outline a plyometrics program for improvin[g] upper body muscular power.
4. Demonstrate proper use of plyometrics by doing the following for each exercise included in Competency 3:
   a. Demonstrate and instruct proper execution of repetitions (form, timing, control).
   b. Explain how and when to adjust the exercise.
   c. Demonstrate ways an athlete can cheat when performing the exercise.
   d. Outline safety factors for the athlete and yourself.
   e. Demonstrate how to record results of this type of therapeutic exercise session.
5. Outline a plyometrics program for improving lower body muscular power.
6. Demonstrate proper use of plyometrics by doing the following for each exercise included in Competency 5:
   a. Demonstrate and instruct proper execution of repetitions (form, timing, control).
   b. Explain how and when to adjust the exercise.
   c. Demonstrate ways an athlete can cheat when performing the exercise.

d. Outline safety factors for the athlete and yourself.

e. De... ...lts of this ...on.

Throwing ball into tramp
Jumping pushups
Jumping to box
Tuck Jump
Bounding

...se causes ...reatest risk of ...y
... Intensity
... 2x a week
...take time to ...ach technique

...s by re-...ing peer ...als per-...ies with ...ssionals, ...demon-...y, dem-

Approved by (date and ...

Bosu pushups
dynx disc lunges
dynx disc plank

high risk
high reward

* Need to work all joints

* Incorporate right before functional
90% -> muscles/bones need to be ready

5. Lower body program

    Peer _____

    ACI _____

6. Lower body exercises

    Peer _____

    ACI _____

Comments

Cardiorespiratory Endurance

Objective

Develop and demonstrate the skills necessary to properly use therapeutic exercise to improve cardiorespiratory endurance during sport injury rehabilitation.

Competencies

1. Discuss the role of maintaining and improving cardiorespiratory endurance during sport injury rehabilitation, including when during the rehabilitation process these activities should be performed.

2. Demonstrate proper use of the following therapeutic exercises for maintaining and improving cardiorespiratory endurance:

   Upper body

   a. Upper body ergometer

   b. Stationary bicycle

   c. Stair climber

   d. Aquatics

   Lower body

   e. Bicycle ergometer

   f. Treadmill

   g. Stair climber

   h. Aquatics

   i. Running on a field, court, or track

   by doing each of the following for each exercise:

   - Set up the equipment, if necessary.
   - Position the patient.
   - Stabilize the patient during repetitions.
   - Demonstrate and instruct proper execution of repetitions (form, timing, control).
   - Explain how and when to adjust the exercise.
   - Demonstrate ways an athlete can cheat while performing the exercise.

   - Outline safety factors for the athlete and yourself.
   - Demonstrate how to record results of this type of therapeutic exercise session.
   - Demonstrate and explain maintenance and simple repair procedures for the equipment.

References

Allsen, Harrison, and Vance 1997 (pp. 45-58)

Arnheim and Prentice 2000 (pp. 76-87)

Houglum 2001 (pp. 416, 499)

Prentice 1999a (pp. 134-142)

Mastery and Demonstration

Practice and reinforce these competencies by reviewing your class notes and texts, observing peer teachers and certified/licensed professionals perform the skills, discussing the competencies with peer teachers and certified/licensed professionals, practicing alone and with a peer, and then demonstrating proficiency to a peer teacher. Finally, demonstrate your proficiency to an ACI.

Approved by (date and signature)

1. Background

   Peer _____

   ACI _____

2a. Upper body—bicycle ergometer

   Peer _____

   ACI _____

2b. Upper body—stationary bike

   Peer _____

   ACI _____

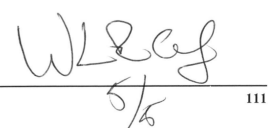

2c. Upper body—stair climber

    Peer_____

    ACI_____

2d. Upper body—aquatics

    Peer_____

    ACI_____

2e. Lower body—bicycle ergometer

    Peer_____

    ACI_____

2f. Lower body—treadmill

    Peer_____

    ACI_____

2g. Lower body—stair climber

    Peer_____

    ACI_____

2h. Lower body—aquatics

    Peer_____

    ACI_____

2i. Lower body—running

    Peer_____

    ACI_____

Comments

Activity-Specific Skills

Objective

Develop and demonstrate the skills necessary to properly use therapeutic exercise to improve activity-specific skills during sport injury rehabilitation.

Competencies

1. Discuss the role of improving activity-specific skills during sport injury rehabilitation, including when during the rehabilitation process these skills should be performed.

2. Demonstrate proper use of the following therapeutic exercises for improving activity-specific skills:

   a. Running—speed

   b. Running—endurance

   c. Striking

   d. Throwing

   e. Catching

   f. Swimming

   g. Two other sport activities of your choosing

   by doing each of the following for each exercise:

   • Set up equipment, if necessary.

   • Position the patient.

   • Stabilize the patient during repetitions.

   • Demonstrate and instruct proper execution of repetitions (form, timing, control).

   • Explain how and when to adjust the exercise.

   • Demonstrate ways an athlete can cheat while performing the exercise.

   • Outline safety factors for the athlete and yourself.

   • Demonstrate how to record results of this type of therapeutic exercise session.

   • Demonstrate and explain maintenance and simple repair procedures for the equipment.

References

Arnheim and Prentice 2000 (pp. 397-400)

Houglum 2001 (pp. 314-337)

Knight 1995 (pp. 46-55)

Prentice 1999a (pp. 266-283)

Tippett and Voight 1995 (pp. 3-18, 45-94)

Mastery and Demonstration

Practice and reinforce these competencies by reviewing your class notes and texts, observing peer teachers and certified/licensed professionals perform the skills, discussing the competencies with peer teachers and certified/licensed professionals, practicing alone and with a peer, and then demonstrating proficiency to a peer teacher. Finally, demonstrate your proficiency to an ACI.

Approved by (date and signature)

1. Background

   Peer _____

   ACI _____

2a. Running—speed

   Peer _____

   ACI _____

2b. Running—endurance

   Peer _____

   ACI _____

2c. Striking

   Peer _____

   ACI _____

2d. Throwing

   Peer _____

   ACI _____

2e. Catching

    Peer _____

    ACI _____

2f. Swimming

    Peer _____

    ACI _____

2g. Choice 1

    Peer _____

    ACI _____

    Choice 2

    Peer _____

    ACI _____

Comments

Oral/Practical Examination 1

Objectives

Demonstrate your mastery of Level 1 and 2 skills and prepare yourself for the NATABOC O/P examination.

Competencies

Complete your program's O/P examination with a score of at least 85%.

References

Individual module references

Mastery and Demonstration

Date taken_____ Score_____

Approved by_____

Reexamination_____ Score_____

Approved by_____

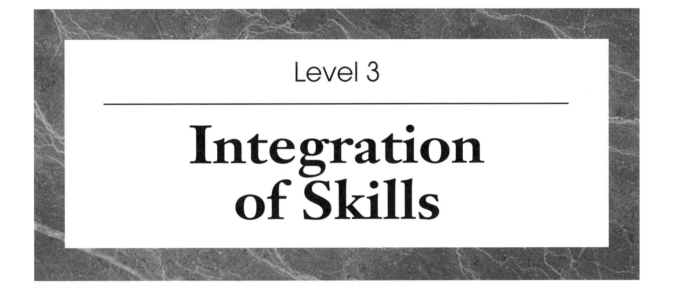

Level 3

Integration of Skills

During Level 3, students will demonstrate their ability to integrate numerous skills to totally manage specific injuries. Although the emphasis in Levels 1 and 2 was on individual skills, the emphasis here is on the injury. Caring for each injury will demonstrate your mastery of related anatomy and the mechanism, assessment, care, rehabilitation, and prevention of that injury.

Clinical experiences will afford athletic training students an opportunity to work with a variety of sports and situations so that they can compare and contrast the injuries that occur in each. There are 30 modules in five groups:

Football Team Experience

Competencies

1. Work a minimum of 4 weeks as a student member of the athletic training staff assigned to a football team.

2. Outline on paper and discuss with your supervisor the following:

a. The organization of athletic training services for the football team. Include the organization (i.e., type of equipment and staff members' functions) of the athletic training clinic and field for practices and games.

b. Proper fitting of all required (by the National Collegiate Athletic Association [NCAA] and the High School Athletic Association) and optional equipment for football. Demonstrate this as well.

c. The skills and activities specific to football that lead to injury.

d. The most common football injuries.

e. Ways to prevent the most common football injuries.

f. NCAA and High School Athletic Association rules about taping and bandaging for games. *cast*

g. NCAA and High School Athletic Association rules about injury care during games.

h. The elements of successful preseason, inseason, and postseason conditioning programs for football. Include activities that develop flexibility, strength, muscular endurance, speed, coordination, agility, power, and cardiorespiratory endurance.

i. The three to five athletes on the team who you feel perform their conditioning exercises most correctly, the three to five who perform them least correctly, and why you chose each.

References

NCAA football rules book (updated yearly)

State High School Association football rules book (most updated yearly)

Mastery and Demonstration

Practice and reinforce these competencies by reviewing your class notes and texts, observing peer teachers and certified/licensed professionals perform the skills, discussing the competencies with peer teachers and certified/licensed professionals, practicing alone and with a peer, and then demonstrating proficiency to a peer teacher. Finally, demonstrate your proficiency to an ACI.

Approved by (date and signature)

1. Assignment completed

Peer _____

ACI _____

2a. Organization

Peer _____

ACI _____

2b. Equipment

Peer _____

ACI _____

2c. Sport skills

Peer _____

ACI _____

2d. Common injuries

Peer _____

ACI _____

2e. Preventing common injuries

Peer _____

ACI _____

2f. Rules about taping   **Comments**

       Peer_____

       ACI_____

2g. Rules about injury care

       Peer_____

       ACI_____

2h. Conditioning programs

       Peer_____

       ACI_____

2i. Athletes

       Peer_____

       ACI_____

Basketball Team Experience

Competencies

1. Work a minimum of 4 weeks as a student member of the athletic training staff assigned to either a men's or women's basketball team.

2. Outline on paper and discuss with your ACI the following:

a. The organization of athletic training services for the basketball team. Include the organization (i.e., type of equipment and staff members' functions) of the athletic training clinic and court for practices and games.

b. Proper fitting of all required (by NCAA and High School Athletic Association) and optional equipment for basketball. Demonstrate this as well.

c. The skills and activities specific to basketball that lead to injury.

d. The most common basketball injuries.

e. Ways to prevent the most common basketball injuries.

f. NCAA and High School Athletic Association rules about taping and bandaging for games.

g. NCAA and High School Athletic Association rules about injury care during games.

h. The elements of successful preseason, in-season, and postseason conditioning programs for basketball. Include activities that develop flexibility, strength, muscular endurance, speed, coordination, agility, power, and cardiorespiratory endurance.

i. The three to five athletes on the team who you feel perform their conditioning exercises most correctly, the three to five who perform them least correctly, and why you chose each.

References

NCAA basketball rules book (updated yearly)

State High School Association basketball rules book (most updated yearly)

Mastery and Demonstration

Practice and reinforce these competencies by reviewing your class notes and texts, observing peer teachers and certified/licensed professionals perform the skills, discussing the competencies with peer teachers and certified/licensed professionals, practicing alone and with a peer, and then demonstrating proficiency to a peer teacher. Finally, demonstrate your proficiency to an ACI.

Approved by (date and signature)

1. Assignment completed

Peer_____

ACI_____

2a. Organization

Peer_____

ACI_____

2b. Equipment

Peer_____

ACI_____

2c. Sport skills

Peer_____

ACI_____

2d. Common injuries

Peer_____

ACI_____

2e. Preventing common injuries

Peer_____

ACI_____

2f. Rules about taping

    Peer _____

    ACI _____

2g. Rules about injury care

    Peer _____

    ACI _____

2h. Conditioning

    Peer _____

    ACI _____

2i. Athletes

    Peer _____

    ACI _____

Comments

Men's Team Sport Experience

Competencies

1. Work a minimum of 4 weeks as a student member of the athletic training staff assigned to a men's team sport (other than football or basketball).

2. Outline on paper and discuss with your ACI the following:

a. The organization of athletic training services for the team. Include the organization (i.e., type of equipment and staff members' functions) of the athletic training clinic and the court or field for practices and games.

b. Proper fitting of all required (by NCAA and High School Athletic Association) and optional equipment for the team. Demonstrate this as well.

c. The skills and activities specific to this sport that lead to injury.

d. The most common injuries in this sport.

e. Ways to prevent the most common injuries in this sport.

f. NCAA and High School Athletic Association rules about taping and bandaging for this sport's contest.

g. NCAA and High School Athletic Association rules about injury care during this sport's contest.

h. Differences (from the athletic training point of view) between this sport and other sports you have worked.

i. The elements of successful preseason, inseason, and postseason conditioning programs for this sport. Include activities that develop flexibility, strength, muscular endurance, speed, coordination, agility, power, and cardiorespiratory endurance.

j. The three to five athletes on the team who you feel perform their conditioning exercises most correctly, the three to five who perform them least correctly, and why you chose each.

References

Certified athletic trainers and coaches assigned to the sport

NCAA rules book for the sport (updated yearly)

State High School Association rules book for the sport (most updated yearly)

Mastery and Demonstration

Practice and reinforce these competencies by reviewing your class notes and texts, observing peer teachers and certified/licensed professionals perform the skills, discussing the competencies with peer teachers and certified/licensed professionals, practicing alone and with a peer, and then demonstrating proficiency to a peer teacher. Finally, demonstrate your proficiency to an ACI.

Approved by (date and signature)

1. Assignment completed

Peer _____

ACI _____

2a. Organization

Peer _____

ACI _____

2b. Equipment

Peer _____

ACI _____

2c. Sport skills

Peer _____

ACI _____

2d. Common injuries

Peer _____

ACI _____

Module X6—Men's Team Sport Experience (continued)

2e. Preventing common injuries   **Comments**

    Peer _____

    ACI _____

2f. Rules about taping

    Peer _____

    ACI _____

2g. Rules about injury care

    Peer _____

    ACI _____

2h. Differences

    Peer _____

    ACI _____

2i. Conditioning

    Peer _____

    ACI _____

2j. Athletes

    Peer _____

    ACI _____

Women's Team Sport Experience

Competencies

1. Work a minimum of 4 weeks as a student member of the athletic training staff assigned to a women's team sport (other than basketball).

2. Outline on paper and discuss with your ACI the following:

a. The organization of athletic training services for the team. Include the organization (i.e., type of equipment and staff members' functions) of the athletic training clinic and the court or field for practices and games.

b. Proper fitting of all required (by NCAA and High School Athletic Association) and optional equipment for the team. Demonstrate this as well.

c. The skills and activities specific to this sport that lead to injury.

d. The most common injuries in this sport.

e. Ways to prevent the most common injuries in this sport.

f. NCAA and High School Athletic Association rules about taping and bandaging for this sport's contest.

g. NCAA and High School Athletic Association rules about injury care during this sport's contest.

h. Differences (from the athletic training point of view) between this sport and other sports you have worked.

i. The elements of successful preseason, in-season, and postseason conditioning programs for this sport. Include activities that develop flexibility, strength, muscular endurance, speed, coordination, agility, power, and cardiorespiratory endurance.

j. The three to five athletes on the team who you feel perform their conditioning exercises most correctly, the three to five who perform them least correctly, and why you chose each.

References

Certified athletic trainers and coaches assigned to the sport

NCAA rules book for the sport (updated yearly)

State High School Association rules book for the sport (most updated yearly)

Mastery and Demonstration

Practice and reinforce these competencies by reviewing your class notes and texts, observing peer teachers and certified/licensed professionals perform the skills, discussing the competencies with peer teachers and certified/licensed professionals, practicing alone and with a peer, and then demonstrating proficiency to a peer teacher. Finally, demonstrate your proficiency to an ACI.

Approved by (date and signature)

1. Assignment completed

Peer_____

ACI_____

2a. Organization

Peer_____

ACI_____

2b. Equipment

Peer_____

ACI_____

2c. Sport skills

Peer_____

ACI_____

2d. Common injuries

Peer_____

ACI_____

2e. Preventing common injuries

    Peer_____

    ACI_____

2f. Rules about taping

    Peer_____

    ACI_____

2g. Rules about injury care

    Peer_____

    ACI_____

2h. Differences

    Peer_____

    ACI_____

2i. Conditioning

    Peer_____

    ACI_____

2j. Athletes

    Peer_____

    ACI_____

Comments

Men's Individual Sport Experience

Competencies

1. Work a minimum of 4 weeks as a student member of the athletic training staff for a men's team that involves individual sport competition (e.g., gymnastics or track and field).

2. Outline on paper and discuss with your ACI the following:

a. The organization of athletic training services for the team. Include the organization (i.e., type of equipment and staff members' functions) of the athletic training clinic and the court or field for practices and games.

b. Proper fitting of all required (by NCAA and High School Athletic Association) and optional equipment for the team. Demonstrate this as well.

c. The skills and activities specific to this sport that lead to injury.

d. The most common injuries in this sport.

e. Ways to prevent the most common injuries in this sport.

f. NCAA and High School Athletic Association rules about taping and bandaging for this sport's contest.

g. NCAA and High School Athletic Association rules about injury care during this sport's contest.

h. Differences (from the athletic training point of view) between this sport and other sports you have worked.

i. The elements of successful preseason, in-season, and postseason conditioning programs for this sport. Include activities that develop flexibility, strength, muscular endurance, speed, coordination, agility, power, and cardiorespiratory endurance.

j. The three to five athletes on the team who you feel perform their conditioning exercises most correctly, the three to five who perform them least correctly, and why you chose each.

References

Certified athletic trainers and coaches assigned to the sport

NCAA rules book for the sport (updated yearly)

State High School Association rules book for the sport (most updated yearly)

Mastery and Demonstration

Practice and reinforce these competencies by reviewing your class notes and texts, observing peer teachers and certified/licensed professionals perform the skills, discussing the competencies with peer teachers and certified/licensed professionals, practicing alone and with a peer, and then demonstrating proficiency to a peer teacher. Finally, demonstrate your proficiency to an ACI.

Approved by (date and signature)

1. Assignment completed

Peer _____

ACI _____

2a. Organization

Peer _____

ACI _____

2b. Equipment

Peer _____

ACI _____

2c. Sport skills

Peer _____

ACI _____

2d. Common injuries

Peer _____

ACI _____

2e. Preventing common injuries   **Comments**

Peer _____

ACI _____

2f. Rules about taping

Peer _____

ACI _____

2g. Rules about injury care

Peer _____

ACI _____

2h. Differences

Peer _____

ACI _____

2i. Conditioning

Peer _____

ACI _____

2j. Athletes

Peer _____

ACI _____

Women's Individual Sport Experience

Competencies

1. Work a minimum of 4 weeks as a student member of the athletic training staff for a women's team that involves individual sport competition (e.g., gymnastics or track and field).

2. Outline on paper and discuss with your ACI the following:

   a. The organization of athletic training services for the team. Include the organization (i.e., type of equipment and staff members' functions) of the athletic training clinic and the court or field for practices and games.

   b. Proper fitting of all required (by NCAA and High School Athletic Association) and optional equipment for the team. Demonstrate this as well.

   c. The skills and activities specific to this sport that lead to injury.

   d. The most common injuries in this sport.

   e. Ways to prevent the most common injuries in this sport.

   f. NCAA and High School Athletic Association rules about taping and bandaging for this sport's contest.

   g. NCAA and High School Athletic Association rules about injury care during this sport's contest.

   h. Differences (from the athletic training point of view) between this sport and other sports you have worked.

   i. The elements of successful preseason, inseason, and postseason conditioning programs for this sport. Include activities that develop flexibility, strength, muscular endurance, speed, coordination, agility, power, and cardiorespiratory endurance.

   j. The three to five athletes on the team who you feel perform their conditioning exercises most correctly, the three to five who perform them least correctly, and why you chose each.

References

Certified athletic trainers and coaches assigned to the sport

NCAA rules book for the sport (updated yearly)

State High School Association rules book for the sport (most updated yearly)

Mastery and Demonstration

Practice and reinforce these competencies by reviewing your class notes and texts, observing peer teachers and certified/licensed professionals perform the skills, discussing the competencies with peer teachers and certified/licensed professionals, practicing alone and with a peer, and then demonstrating proficiency to a peer teacher. Finally, demonstrate your proficiency to an ACI.

Approved by (date and signature)

1. Assignment completed

   Peer _____

   ACI _____

2a. Organization

   Peer _____

   ACI _____

2b. Equipment

   Peer _____

   ACI _____

2c. Sport skills

   Peer _____

   ACI _____

2d. Common injuries

     Peer _____

     ACI _____

2e. Preventing common injuries

     Peer _____

     ACI _____

2f. Rules about taping

     Peer _____

     ACI _____

2g. Rules about injury care

     Peer _____

     ACI _____

2h. Differences

     Peer _____

     ACI _____

2i. Conditioning

     Peer _____

     ACI _____

2j. Athletes

     Peer _____

     ACI _____

Comments

High School Experience

Competencies

1. Work a minimum of 4 weeks as a student member of the athletic training staff for a high school.

2. Outline on paper and discuss with your ACI the following:

   a. The organization of athletic training services for the school. Include the organization (i.e., type of equipment and staff members' functions) of the athletic training clinic and the court or field for practices and games.

   b. Role of parents and personal physicians in care of the juvenile athlete's injuries and illnesses.

   c. Differences between juveniles and adults in how they deal with pain.

   d. Injuries and illnesses that are more prevalent in juveniles than in college athletes.

   e. Injuries and illnesses that are less prevalent in juveniles than in college athletes.

   f. Time for treating injuries.

   g. Differences (from the athletic training point of view) between high school and college athletics.

References

High school certified athletic trainers and coaches

State High School Association rules book for the sport (most updated yearly)

Mastery and Demonstration

Practice and reinforce these competencies by reviewing your class notes and texts, observing peer teachers and certified/licensed professionals perform the skills, discussing the competencies with peer teachers and certified/licensed professionals, practicing alone and with a peer, and then demonstrating proficiency to a peer teacher. Finally, demonstrate your proficiency to an ACI.

Approved by (date and signature)

1. Assignment completed

   Peer _____

   ACI _____

2a. Organization

   Peer _____

   ACI _____

2b. Roles

   Peer _____

   ACI _____

2c. Differences between juveniles and adults

   Peer _____

   ACI _____

2d. Common injuries in juveniles

   Peer _____

   ACI _____

2e. Less common injuries in juveniles

   Peer _____

   ACI _____

2f. Treatment time

   Peer _____

   ACI _____

2g. Differences

   Peer _____

   ACI _____

Comments

Sports Medicine Clinic Experience

Competencies

1. Work a minimum of 4 weeks as a student member of the athletic training staff in a sports medicine clinic.

2. Outline on paper and discuss with your ACI the following:

   a. The organization of athletic training services of the clinic. Include the organization (i.e., type of equipment and staff members' functions) in the clinic and any high school or college outreach services provided.

   b. The most common injuries seen in the clinic.

   c. Differences between working in a sports medicine clinic and a college or high school based athletic training department.

References

Clinic staff

Mastery and Demonstration

Obtain the signature of an ACI when you have completed this module.

Approved by (date and signature)

1. Assignment completed

   Peck _____

   ACI _____

2a. Organization

   Peck _____

   ACI _____

2b. Common injuries

   Peck _____

   ACI _____

2c. Differences

   Peer _____

   ACI _____

Comments

Supervise/Teach Level 2 Students

Objective

Teach Level 2 skills, assess mastery of those skills by Level 2 students, and deepen your own understanding and mastery of those skills.

Competencies

1. Peer teach at least four different Level 2 students and at least 15 Level 2 modules. This includes reviewing material with the students, offering suggestions and corrections as necessary as they practice the skills, and then assessing their mastery of the skill when appropriate. Students must practice the skills long enough that they become proficient with them before assessment. Refer often to references and teaching aids.

2. Discuss your peer teaching experience with a faculty athletic trainer or clinical instructor.

References

Your athletic training department library and the references to individual Level 2 modules

Mastery and Demonstration

1. Record your peer teaching experiences in the spaces provided:

Name of Student	Module	Review Date	Approval Date
1.			
2.			
3.			
4.			
5.			
6.			
7.			
8.			
9.			
10.			
11.			
12.			
13.			
14.			
15.			
16.			
17.			
18.			

Name of Student	Module	Review Date	Assessment Date
19. _____	_____	_____	_____
20. _____	_____	_____	_____
21. _____	_____	_____	_____
22. _____	_____	_____	_____
23. _____	_____	_____	_____
24. _____	_____	_____	_____
25. _____	_____	_____	_____
26. _____	_____	_____	_____
27. _____	_____	_____	_____
28. _____	_____	_____	_____
29. _____	_____	_____	_____
30. _____	_____	_____	_____

2. Task completed and discussed (date)

_____

Approved by

_____

Comments

Administer O/P Examination 1

Objective

Deepen your understanding and mastery of Levels 1 and 2 skills by examining others.

Competency

Help your program director examine Level 2 students by serving as an examiner for at least five different O/P examinations.

Person examined	Date
1.	
2.	
3.	
4.	
5.	
6.	
7.	
8.	
9.	
10.	
11.	
12.	
13.	
14.	
15.	

Completion

Peer _____

ACI _____

Comments

Surgical Observation

Objective

Develop an appreciation for what athletes go through during surgery. Note: J modules can be completed simultaneously with this module.

Competencies

1. Observe two different surgical procedures. With each, discuss with a physician, surgical nurse, or technician the presurgical preparation of the patient and the procedures that will be followed for the 12 to 24 hours after surgery.

2. Within 48 hours of the surgery (the sooner the better), discuss the surgery with a peer teacher. Include in this discussion the rehabilitation procedures that this patient probably will follow.

Completion

Surgery 1:

Athlete _____

Procedure _____

Date _____

Physician _____

Approved by (date and signature)

ACI _____

Surgery 2:

Athlete _____

Procedure _____

Date _____

Physician _____

Approved by (date and signature)

ACI _____

Comments

LEVEL 3

Module J1
Specific Injury Management

Foot Injury Management

Objective

Develop and demonstrate the skills necessary to properly evaluate, care for, rehabilitate, and prevent foot injuries.

Anatomy and Conditions for This Module

A. Bones and Prominent Bony Features

- Calcaneus
- Talus
- Cuboid
- Navicular
- Cuneiforms
- Metatarsals
  - Styloid process of fifth heads
  - Phalanges
  - Sesamoids

B. Articulations

- Subtalar
- Transverse tarsal
- Metatarsal-phalangeal (MP)
- Interphalangeal (PIP and DIP)

C. Ligaments

- Long plantar
- Lateral retinaculum

D. Muscles

- Anterior tibialis
- Flexor hallicus longus
- Flexor digitorum longus
- Posterior tibialis
- Extensor hallicus longus
- Extensor digitorum longus
- Peroneus longus
- Peroneus brevis
- Peroneus tertius

- Gastrocnemius
- Soleus

E. Other Structures

- Peroneal nerve (entire course)
- Tibial nerve (entire course)
- Pedal pulse

F. Special Tests

- Compression test (e.g., Pott's fracture)
- Percussion test
- Tinel's sign
- Weight-bearing versus non-weight-bearing alignment
- Gait analysis compression test (e.g., Pott's fracture)

G. Injuries and Conditions

1 • Ingrown toenail (paronychia)
2 • Bunions
3 • Calluses and corns
4 • Blisters
5 • Neuroma
6 • Plantarflexed first ray
7 • Mallet toe
8 • Claw toes
9 • Sprained hallux
10 • Sprained digit
11 • Exostosis
12 • Tarsal tunnel syndrome
13 • Apophysitis (Sever's disease)
14 • Dislocation or subluxation
15 • Forefoot varus/valgus
16 • Equinus deformity
17 • Pes cavus/planus
18 • Rearfoot (hindfoot) varus/valgus
19 • Hallux rigidus
20 • Hallux valgus

- 21 Morton's foot syndrome
- 22 Arch strains
- 23 Plantar fasciitis
- 24 Heel bruise
- 25 Bursitis
- 26 Tendinitis
- 27 Tenosynovitis
- 28 Fracture
- 29 Stress fracture
- 30 Avulsion fracture
- 31 Sinis tarsi syndrome

Competencies

Note: All procedures must be performed.

Anatomical Review and Assessment of Structural Integrity

1. Name and palpate each bone and bony structure in list A. Also, tell what differences you would expect to feel if the bone was fractured.

2. Palpate or draw the joint line for each articulation in list B. Then perform active and passive joint ROM tests using both qualitative and quantitative techniques (e.g., tape measure, goniometer, and inclinometer). Record results of these tests using accepted forms and procedures.

3. Using surface anatomy, palpate or draw the origins and course of each ligament in list C.

4. Using surface anatomy, palpate the origin, insertion, and course of each muscle in list D. Also, tell the major function of each muscle.

5. Using surface anatomy, palpate each structure in list E.

Injury Assessment

6. Obtain the medical history of an athlete with a suspected foot injury.

7. Demonstrate proper administration and interpretation of the special tests in list F.

8. Demonstrate how you would observe and identify the clinical signs and symptoms associated with the injuries and conditions in list G.

9. Explain and demonstrate the mechanisms by which each injury in list G occurs. Name the three sports in which each injury is most likely to occur and explain any differences among the injury occurrences and mechanisms in those sports.

10. Demonstrate appropriate sensory, circulatory, and neurological tests for the injuries in list G.

11. Palpate and assess the integrity of the bones and soft tissues associated with each injury in list G.

12. Perform special tests to assess the integrity of the joints involved in each injury in list G and explain how you would interpret these tests.

13. Demonstrate the use of manual muscle testing and other tests as appropriate to assess the flexibility and strength of the muscles associated with each injury in list G.

14. Demonstrate functional and activity-specific tests to determine the integrity of each structure involved in each injury in list G.

Injury Management

15. Explain and demonstrate the appropriate immediate care procedures for each injury in list G. Explain the objectives and criteria for progressing for each step in the procedure.

16. Demonstrate a complete rehabilitation program for each injury in list G. As you proceed, explain the objectives and procedures of each step in the program. Explain the measurement criteria for advancing from one step to another.

Risk Management

17. Using pictures or illustrations, explain the objectives and procedures of prophylactic taping, padding, and bandaging, as appropriate, for the injuries in list G.

18. Demonstrate or explain procedures for preventing each injury in list G.

References

AAOS 1999 (pp. 490-523)

Anderson, Hall, and Martin 2000 (pp. 483-528)

Arnheim and Prentice 2000 (pp. 446-481)

Houglum 2001 (pp. 757-833)

Magee 1997 (pp. 559-666)

Shultz, Houglum, and Perrin 2000 (pp. 229-267)

Starkey and Ryan 2002 (pp. 87-135)

Philip Tayer 4.5/5 2-18-10

Mastery and Demonstration

Practice and reinforce these competencies by reviewing your class notes and texts, observing peer teachers and certified/licensed professionals perform the skills, discussing the competencies with peer teachers and certified/licensed professionals, practicing alone and with a peer, and then demonstrating proficiency to a peer teacher. Finally, demonstrate your proficiency to an ACI.

Approved by (date and signature):

1. Bones

Peer _____

ACI _____

2. Joints

Peer _____

ACI _____

3. Ligaments

Peer _____

ACI _____

4. Muscles

Peer _____

ACI _____

5. Other structures

Peer _____

ACI _____

6. History

Peer _____

ACI _____

7. Special Tests

- Compression test

Peer _____

ACI _____

- Percussion test

Peer _____

ACI _____

- Tinel's sign

Peer _____

ACI _____

- Weight-bearing vs. non-weight-bearing

Peer _____

ACI _____

- Gait analysis

Peer _____

ACI _____

8-18. Complete competencies 8-18 for the injuries or conditions in list G:

- Ingrown toenail

Peer _____

ACI _____

- Bunions

Peer _____

ACI _____

- Calluses and corns

Peer _____

ACI _____

- Blisters

Peer _____

ACI _____

- Neuroma

Peer _____

ACI _____

- Plantarflexed first ray

Peer _____

ACI _____

- Mallet toe

Peer _____

ACI _____

- Claw toes

Peer _____

ACI _____

- Sprained hallux

Peer _____

ACI _____

- Sprained digit

  Peer_____

  ACI_____

- Exostosis

  Peer_____

  ACI_____

- Tarsal tunnel syndrome

  Peer_____

  ACI_____

- Apophysitis

  Peer_____

  ACI_____

- Dislocation or subluxation

  Peer_____

  ACI_____

- Forefoot varus/valgus

  Peer_____

  ACI_____

- Equinus deformity

  Peer_____

  ACI_____

- Pes cavus/planus

  Peer_____

  ACI_____

- Rearfoot (hindfoot) varus/valgus

  Peer_____

  ACI_____

- Hallux rigidus

  Peer_____

  ACI_____

- Hallux valgus

  Peer_____

  ACI_____

- Morton's foot syndrome

  Peer_____

  ACI_____

- Arch strains

  Peer_____

  ACI_____

- Plantar fasciitis

  Peer_____

  ACI_____

- Heel bruise

  Peer_____

  ACI_____

- Bursitis

  Peer_____

  ACI_____

- Tendinitis

  Peer_____

  ACI_____

- Tenosynovitis

  Peer_____

  ACI_____

- Fracture

  Peer_____

  ACI_____

- Stress fracture

  Peer_____

  ACI_____

- Avulsion fracture

  Peer_____

  ACI_____

- Sinus tarsi syndrome

  Peer_____

  ACI_____

Ankle Injury Management

Objective

Develop and demonstrate the skills necessary to properly evaluate, care for, rehabilitate, and prevent ankle injuries.

Anatomy and Conditions for This Module

A. Bones and Prominent Bony Features

- Calcaneus
- Talus
- Cuboid
- Navicular
- Cuneiforms
- Tibia
- Fibula

B. Articulations

- Ankle mortice
- Distal tibiofibular
- Subtalar
- Transverse tarsal

C. Ligaments

- Anterior talofibular
- Calcaneofibular
- Posterior talofibular
- Distal anterior tibiofibular
- Distal posterior tibiofibular
- Deltoid
- Peroneal retinaculum

D. Muscles

- Anterior tibialis
- Flexor hallicus longus
- Flexor digitorum longus
- Posterior tibialis
- Extensor hallicus longus
- Extensor digitorum longus
- Peroneus longus
- Peroneus brevis
- Peroneus tertius
- Gastrocnemius
- Soleus

E. Other Structures

- Anterior tibial artery
- Deep peroneal nerve
- Superficial peroneal nerve
- Posterior tibial

F. Special Tests

- Anterior drawer test
- Talar tilt test
- Kleiger's test—ankle
- Tap test

G. Injuries and Conditions

1. First-degree ankle sprain
2. Second-degree ankle sprain
3. Third-degree ankle sprain
4. Sprain-dislocation
5. Anterior tibial strain
6. Peroneal strain
7. Fracture
8. Stress fracture
9. Avulsion fracture

Competencies

Note: All procedures must be performed.

Anatomical Review and Assessment of Structural Integrity

1. Name and palpate each bone and bony structure in list A. Also, tell what differences you would expect to feel if the bone was fractured.

2. Palpate or draw the joint line for each articulation in list B. Then perform active and pas-

sive joint ROM tests using both qualitative and quantitative techniques (e.g., tape measure, goniometer, and inclinometer). Record results of these tests using accepted forms and procedures.

3. Using surface anatomy, palpate or draw the origins and course of each ligament in list C.

4. Using surface anatomy, palpate the origin, insertion, and course of each muscle in list D. Also, tell the major function of each muscle.

5. Using surface anatomy, palpate each structure in list E.

Injury Assessment

6. Obtain the medical history of an athlete with a suspected ankle injury.

7. Demonstrate proper administration and interpretation of the special tests in list F.

8. Demonstrate how you would observe and identify the clinical signs and symptoms associated with the injuries and conditions in list G.

9. Explain and demonstrate the mechanisms by which each injury in list G occurs. Name the three sports in which each injury is most likely to occur and explain any differences among the injury occurrences and mechanisms in those sports.

10. Demonstrate appropriate sensory, circulatory, and neurological tests for the injuries in list G.

11. Palpate and assess the integrity of the bones and soft tissues associated with each injury in list G.

12. Perform special tests to assess the integrity of the joints involved in each injury in list G and explain how you would interpret these tests.

13. Demonstrate the use of manual muscle testing and other tests as appropriate to assess the flexibility and strength of the muscles associated with each injury in list G.

14. Demonstrate functional and activity-specific tests to determine the integrity of each structure involved in each injury in list G.

Injury Management

15. Explain and demonstrate the appropriate immediate care procedures for each injury in list

G. Explain the objectives and criteria for progressing for each step in the procedure.

16. Demonstrate a complete rehabilitation program for each injury in list G. As you proceed, explain the objectives and procedures of each step in the program. Explain the measurement criteria for advancing from one step to another.

Risk Management

17. Using pictures or illustrations, explain the objectives and procedures of prophylactic taping, padding, and bandaging, as appropriate, for the injuries in list G.

18. Demonstrate or explain procedures for preventing each injury in list G.

References

AAOS 1999 (pp. 490-523)

Anderson, Hall, and Martin 2000 (pp. 483-528)

Arnheim and Prentice 2000 (pp. 482-497, 507-514)

Houglum 2001 (pp. 757-833)

Magee 1997 (pp. 599-666)

Shultz, Houglum, and Perrin 2000 (pp. 229-267)

Starkey and Ryan 2002 (pp. 136-185)

Mastery and Demonstration

Practice and reinforce these competencies by reviewing your class notes and texts, observing peer teachers and certified/licensed professionals perform the skills, discussing the competencies with peer teachers and certified/licensed professionals, practicing alone and with a peer, and then demonstrating proficiency to a peer teacher. Finally, demonstrate your proficiency to an ACI.

Approved by (date and signature)

1. Bones

   Peer _____

   ACI _____

2. Joints

   Peer _____

   ACI _____

Module J2—Ankle Injury Management (continued)

3. Ligaments

Peer _____

ACI _____

4. Muscles

Peer _____

ACI _____

5. Other structures

Peer _____

ACI _____

6. History

Peer _____

ACI _____

7. Special Tests

- Anterior drawer test

Peer _____

ACI _____

- Talar tilt test

Peer _____

ACI _____

- Kleiger's test—ankle

Peer _____

ACI _____

- Tap test

Peer _____

ACI _____

8-18. Complete competencies 8-18 for the injuries or conditions in list G:

- First-degree ankle sprain

Peer _____

ACI _____

- Second-degree ankle sprain

Peer _____

ACI _____

- Third-degree ankle sprain

Peer _____

ACI _____

- Sprain-dislocation

Peer _____

ACI _____

- Anterior tibial strain

Peer _____

ACI _____

- Peroneal strain

Peer _____

ACI _____

- Fracture

Peer _____

ACI _____

- Stress fracture

Peer _____

ACI _____

- Avulsion fracture

Peer _____

ACI _____

Comments

Lower Leg Injury Management

Objective

Develop and demonstrate the skills necessary to properly evaluate, care for, rehabilitate, and prevent lower leg injuries.

Anatomy and Conditions for This Module

A. Bones and Prominent Bony Features

- Tibia
  - Anterior border
  - Medial condyle
  - Lateral condyle
  - Gerdy's tubercle
  - Patellar tubercle
  - Malleolus
- Fibula
  - Head
  - Shaft
  - Malleolus

B. Articulations

- Proximal tibiofibular
- Distal tibiofibular

C. Ligaments

- Interosseous ligament

D. Muscles

- Anterior tibialis ✓
- Posterior tibialis ✓
- Flexor hallicus longus ✓
- Flexor digitorum longus ✓
- Extensor hallicus longus ✓
- Extensor digitorum longus ✓
- Peroneus longus ✓
- Peroneus tertius
- Gastrocnemius ✓
- Soleus ✓

E. Other Structures

- Common peroneal nerve (entire course)
- Pedal pulse

F. Special Tests

- Homan's sign
- Thompson's test

G. Injuries and Conditions

1. Achilles tendon strain/rupture
2. Achilles bursitis and tenosynovitis
3. Anterior shin splints
4. Posterior shin splints
5. Compartment syndrome
6. Muscular strains and rupture
7. Contusion
8. Peroneal nerve contusion
9. Fracture
10. Stress fracture
11. Tibial stress syndrome
12. Fasciitis
13. Osteochondritis dissecans
14. Deep vein thrombosis

Competencies

Note: All procedures must be performed.

Anatomical Review and Assessment of Structural Integrity

1. Name and palpate each bone and bony structure in list A. Also, tell what differences you would expect to feel if the bone was fractured.

2. Palpate or draw the joint line for each articulation in list B. Then perform active and passive joint ROM tests using both qualitative and quantitative techniques (e.g., tape measure, goniometer, and inclinometer). Record results of these tests using accepted forms and procedures.

3. Using surface anatomy, palpate or draw the origins and course of each ligament in list C.

4. Using surface anatomy, palpate the origin, insertion, and course of each muscle in list D. Also, tell the major function of each muscle.

5. Using surface anatomy, palpate each structure in list E.

Injury Assessment

6. Obtain the medical history of an athlete with a suspected lower leg injury.

7. Demonstrate proper administration and interpretation of the special tests in list F.

8. Demonstrate how you would observe and identify the clinical signs and symptoms associated with the injuries and conditions in list G.

9. Explain and demonstrate the mechanisms by which each injury in list G occurs. Name the three sports in which each injury is most likely to occur and explain any differences among the injury occurrences and mechanisms in those sports.

10. Demonstrate appropriate sensory, circulatory, and neurological tests for the injuries in list G.

11. Palpate and assess the integrity of the bones and soft tissues associated with each injury in list G.

12. Perform special tests to assess the integrity of the joints involved in each injury in list G and explain how you would interpret these tests.

13. Demonstrate the use of manual muscle testing and other tests as appropriate to assess the flexibility and strength of the muscles associated with each injury in list G.

14. Demonstrate functional and activity-specific tests to determine the integrity of each structure involved in each injury in list G.

Injury Management

15. Explain and demonstrate the appropriate immediate care procedures for each injury in list G. Explain the objectives and criteria for progressing for each step in the procedure.

16. Demonstrate a complete rehabilitation program for each injury in list G. As you proceed, explain the objectives and procedures of each step in the program. Explain the measurement criteria for advancing from one step to another.

Risk Management

17. Using pictures or illustrations, explain the objectives and procedures of prophylactic taping, padding, and bandaging, as appropriate, for the injuries in list G.

18. Demonstrate or explain procedures for preventing each injury in list G.

References

AAOS 1999 (pp. 490-523)

Anderson, Hall, and Martin 2000 (pp. 483-528)

Arnheim and Prentice 2000 (pp. 483-491, 497-514)

Houglum 2001 (pp. 757-833)

Magee 1997 (pp. 599-666)

Shultz, Houglum, and Perrin 2000 (pp. 229-267)

Starkey and Ryan 2002 (pp. 86-126)

Mastery and Demonstration

Practice and reinforce these competencies by reviewing your class notes and texts, observing peer teachers and certified/licensed professionals perform the skills, discussing the competencies with peer teachers and certified/licensed professionals, practicing alone and with a peer, and then demonstrating proficiency to a peer teacher. Finally demonstrate your proficiency to an ACI.

Approved by (date and signature)

1. Bones

Peer _____

ACI _____

2. Joints

Peer _____

ACI _____

3. Ligaments

Peer _____

ACI _____

4. Muscles

Peer _____

ACI _____

5. Other structures

Peer _____

ACI _____

6. History

Peer _____

ACI _____

7. Special Tests

- Homan's sign

    Peer _____

    ACI _____

- Thompson's test

    Peer _____

    ACI _____

8-18. Complete competencies 8-18 for the injuries or conditions in list G:

- Achilles strain

    Peer _____

    ACI _____

- Achilles bursitis

    Peer _____

    ACI _____

- Shin splints—anterior

    Peer _____

    ACI _____

- Shin splints—posterior

    Peer _____

    ACI _____

- Compartment syndrome

    Peer _____

    ACI _____

- Muscular strain

    Peer _____

    ACI _____

- Contusion

    Peer _____

    ACI _____

- Peroneal nerve

    Peer _____

    ACI _____

- Fracture

    Peer _____

    ACI _____

- Stress fracture

    Peer _____

    ACI _____

- Tibial stress syndrome

    Peer _____

    ACI _____

- Fasciitis

    Peer _____

    ACI _____

- Osteochondritis

    Peer _____

    ACI _____

- Deep vein thrombosis

    Peer _____

    ACI _____

Comments

Knee Injury Management

Objective

Develop and demonstrate the skills necessary to properly evaluate, care for, rehabilitate, and prevent knee injuries.

Anatomy and Conditions for This Module

A. Bones and Prominent Bony Features

- Femur
  - Condyles
  - Epicondyles
- Tibia
  - Medial condyle
  - Lateral condyle
  - Gerdy's tubercle
- Fibula
  - Head
- Patella

B. Articulations

- Medial tibiofemoral
- Lateral tibiofemoral
- Superior tibiofibular
- Patellotibial

C. Ligaments

- Lateral capsular
- Lateral collateral
- Medial capsular (deep collateral)
- Posterior fibers
- Middle fibers
- Anterior fibers
- Medial collateral (superficial collateral)
- Anterior cruciate (ACL)
- Posterior cruciate (PCL)
- Quadriceps tendon
- Patellar

D. Muscles

- ✓ Biceps femoris (long and short heads)
- ✓ Semitendinosus
- ✓ Semimembranosus
- ✓ Rectus femoris
- ✓ Vastus medialis
- ✓ Vastus intermedius
- ✓ Vastus lateralis
- ✓ Sartorius
- ✓ Tensor fasciae latae
- Iliotibial band
- Gracilis
- ✓ Gastrocnemius (medial and lateral heads)
- ✓ Popliteus

E. Other Structures

- Common peroneal nerve
- Popliteal artery
- Suprapatellar bursa
- Patellar bursa
- Infrapatellar fat pad
- Infrapatellar bursa
- Superficial bursa

F. Special Tests

- Tibiofemoral alignment (e.g., genu recurvatum, genu valgum, genu varum)
- Patellar alignment (e.g., patella alta, patella baja, squinting patella, Q angle)
- Patellar glide, tilt, and rotation
- Valgus stress test
- Varus stress test
- Lachman's test
- Anterior drawer test
- Posterior drawer test
- Posterior sag sign Godfeys
- Slocum's test

- Hughston's test – PCL
- Lateral pivot shift maneuver
- McMurray's test
- Apley's compression and distraction test
- Patellar grind test
- Patellar apprehension test
- Sweep test
- Ballottable patella

G. Injuries and Conditions Duc 3/29

- 1. Torn medial meniscus 233 · 633
- 2. Torn lateral meniscus 233
- 3. ACL sprain 221 · 629
- 4. PCL sprain 222 · 632
- 5. Medial collateral (MCL) sprain (superficial) 218 · 626
- 6. MCL sprain (deep) 218
- 7. Lateral collateral (LCL) sprain 219 · 629
- 8. Anteromedial rotary instability (AMRI)
- 9. Anterolateral rotary instability (ALRI)
- 10. Bursitis 264 · 638
- 11. Capsular contusion
- 12. Contused vastus medialis
- 13. Patellofemoral joint pain · 643
- 14. Patellar tendinitis 262 · 645
- 15. Patellar tendinosis
- 16. Patellar tenosynovitis
- 17. Fractured patella · 638
- 18. Baker's cyst
- 19. Synovial plica 264 · 634
- 20. Hyperextended knee
- 21. Osgood-Schlatter disease 267 · 644
- 22. Iliotibial band syndrome 235 · 646
- 23. Distal hamstring strain
- 24. Chondromalacia patella · 641
- 25. Patellar dislocation and subluxation 260 · 639
- 26. Fat pad contusion · 640
- 27. Fracture
- 28. Osteochondritis dissecans · 635
- 29. Patellar tendon rupture 262 · 646
- 30. Peroneal nerve contusion or palsy · 637
- 31. Tendinitis
- 32. Tibial torsion

Competencies

Note: All procedures must be performed.

Anatomical Review and Assessment of Structural Integrity

1. Name and palpate each bone and bony structure in list A. Also, tell what differences you would expect to feel if the bone was fractured.

2. Palpate or draw the joint line for each articulation in list B. Then perform active and passive joint ROM tests using both qualitative and quantitative techniques (e.g., tape measure, goniometer, and inclinometer). Record results of these tests using accepted forms and procedures.

3. Using surface anatomy, palpate or draw the origins and course of each ligament in list C.

4. Using surface anatomy, palpate the origin, insertion, and course of each muscle in list D. Also, tell the major function of each muscle.

5. Using surface anatomy, palpate each structure in list E.

Injury Assessment

6. Obtain the medical history of an athlete with a suspected knee injury.

7. Demonstrate proper administration and interpretation of the special tests in list F.

8. Demonstrate how you would observe and identify the clinical signs and symptoms associated with the injuries and conditions in list G.

9. Explain and demonstrate the mechanisms by which each injury in list G occurs. Name the three sports in which each injury is most likely to occur and explain any differences among the injury occurrences and mechanisms in those sports.

10. Demonstrate appropriate sensory, circulatory, and neurological tests for the injuries in list G.

11. Palpate and assess the integrity of the bones and soft tissues associated with each injury in list G.

12. Perform special tests to assess the integrity of the joints involved in each injury in list G and explain how you would interpret these tests.

3/31/10

13. Demonstrate the use of manual muscle testing and other tests as appropriate to assess the flexibility and strength of the muscles associated with each injury in list G.

14. Demonstrate functional and activity-specific tests to determine the integrity of each structure involved in each injury in list G.

Injury Management

15. Explain and demonstrate the appropriate immediate care procedures for each injury in list G. Explain the objectives and criteria for progressing for each step in the procedure.

16. Demonstrate a complete rehabilitation program for each injury in list G. As you proceed, explain the objectives and procedures of each step in the program. Explain the measurement criteria for advancing from one step to another.

Risk Management

17. Using pictures or illustrations, explain the objectives and procedures of prophylactic taping, padding, and bandaging, as appropriate, for the injuries in list G.

18. Demonstrate or explain procedures for preventing each injury in list G.

References

AAOS 1999 (pp. 436-487)

Anderson, Hall, and Martin 2000 (pp. 431-482)

Arnheim and Prentice 2000 (pp. 515-564)

Houglum 2001 (pp. 835-903)

Magee 1997 (pp. 506-591)

Shultz, Houglum, and Perrin 2000 (pp. 269-309)

Starkey and Ryan 2002 (pp. 186-270)

Mastery and Demonstration

Practice and reinforce these competencies by reviewing your class notes and texts, observing peer teachers and certified/licensed professionals perform the skills, discussing the competencies with peer teachers and certified/licensed professionals, practicing alone and with a peer, and then demonstrating proficiency to a peer teacher. Finally, demonstrate your proficiency to an ACI.

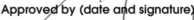

Approved by (date and signature)

1. Bones

   Peer _____

   ACI _____

2. Joints

   Peer _____

   ACI _____

3. Ligaments

   Peer _____

   ACI _____

4. Muscles

   Peer _____

   ACI _____

5. Other structures

   Peer _____

   ACI _____

6. History

   Peer _____

   ACI _____

7. Special Tests

   - Tibiofemoral alignment

     Peer _____

     ACI _____

   - Patellar alignment

     Peer _____

     ACI _____

   - Patellar glide, tilt, and rotation

     Peer _____

     ACI _____

   - Valgus stress test

     Peer _____

     ACI _____

   - Varus stress test

     Peer _____

     ACI _____

Module J4—Knee Injury Management (continued)

- Lachman's test

  Peer _____ *MJG*

  ACI _____

- Anterior drawer test

  Peer _____ *MJG*

  ACI _____

- Posterior drawer test

  Peer _____ *MJG*

  ACI _____

- Posterior sag sign

  Peer _____ *MJG*

  ACI _____

- Slocum's test

  Peer _____ *MJG*

  ACI _____

- Hughston's test

  Peer _____ *MJG*

  ACI _____

- Lateral pivot shift maneuver

  Peer _____ *MJG*

  ACI _____

- McMurray's test

  Peer _____ *MJG*

  ACI _____

- Apley's compression and distraction test

  Peer _____ *MJG*

  ACI _____

- Patellar grind test

  Peer _____ *MJG*

  ACI _____

- Patellar apprehension test

  Peer _____ *MJG*

  ACI _____

- Sweep test

  Peer _____ *MJG*

  ACI _____

- Ballottable patella

  Peer _____ *MJG*

  ACI _____

8-18. Complete competencies 8-18 for the following injuries or conditions in list G:

- Torn medial meniscus

  Peer _____

  ACI _____

- Torn lateral meniscus

  Peer _____

  ACI _____

- ACL sprain

  Peer _____

  ACI _____

- PCL sprain

  Peer _____

  ACI _____

- MCL sprain—superficial

  Peer _____

  ACI _____

- MCL sprain—deep

  Peer _____

  ACI _____

- LCL sprain

  Peer _____

  ACI _____

- AMRI

  Peer _____

  ACI _____

- ALRI

  Peer _____

  ACI _____

- Bursitis

  Peer _____

  ACI _____

- Capsular contusion

  Peer _____

  ACI _____

- Contused vastus medialis

  Peer _____

  ACI _____

- Patellofemoral joint pain

  Peer _____

  ACI _____

- Patellar tendinitis

  Peer _____

  ACI _____

- Patellar tendinosis

  Peer _____

  ACI _____

- Patellar tenosynovitis

  Peer _____

  ACI _____

- Fractured patella

  Peer _____

  ACI _____

- Baker's cyst

  Peer _____

  ACI _____

- Synovial plica

  Peer _____

  ACI _____

- Hyperextended knee

  Peer _____

  ACI _____

- Osgood-Schlatter disease

  Peer _____

  ACI _____

- Iliotibial band syndrome

  Peer _____

  ACI _____

- Distal hamstring strain

  Peer _____

  ACI _____

- Chondromalacia patella

  Peer _____

  ACI _____

- Patellar dislocation and subluxation

  Peer _____

  ACI _____

- Fat pad contusion

  Peer _____

  ACI _____

- Fracture

  Peer _____

  ACI _____

- Osteochondritis dissecans

  Peer _____

  ACI _____

- Patellar tendon rupture

  Peer _____

  ACI _____

- Peroneal nerve contusion

  Peer _____

  ACI _____

- Tendinitis

  Peer _____

  ACI _____

- Tibial torsion

  Peer _____

  ACI _____

Comments

LEVEL 3

Module J5
Specific Injury Management

Thigh Injury Management

Objective

Develop and demonstrate the skills necessary to properly evaluate, care for, rehabilitate, and prevent thigh injuries.

Anatomy and Conditions for This Module

A. Bones and Prominent Bony Features

- Femur
  - Condyles
  - Epicondyles
- Tibia
  - Medial condyle
  - Lateral condyle
  - Gerdy's tubercle
  - Patellar tubercle
- Fibula
  - Head
- Patella

B. Articulations

- Medial tibiofemoral
- Lateral tibiofemoral
- Patellotibial

C. Muscles

- Biceps femoris (long and short heads) ✓
- Semitendinosus ✓
- Semimembranosus ✓
- Rectus femoris ✓
- Vastus medialis ✓
- Vastus intermedius ✓
- Vastus lateralis ✓
- Sartorius ✓
- Hip adductor group
- Tensor fasciae latae ✓

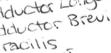

Adductor Magnus
Adductor Longus
Adductor Brevis
Gracilis
Pactineus

- Iliotibial band
- Gracilis

D. Other Structures

- Sciatic nerve
- Femoral nerve

E. Injuries and Conditions

- Quadriceps contusion
- Quadriceps strain
- Hamstring strain
- Femoral fracture
- Myositis ossificans
- Patellar tendon rupture

Competencies

Note: All procedures must be performed.

Anatomical Review and Assessment of Structural Integrity

1. Name and palpate each bone and bony structure in list A. Also, tell what differences you would expect to feel if the bone was fractured.

2. Palpate or draw the joint line for each articulation in list B. Then perform active and passive joint ROM tests using both qualitative and quantitative techniques (e.g., tape measure, goniometer, and inclinometer). Record results of these tests using accepted forms and procedures.

3. Using surface anatomy, palpate the origin, insertion, and course of each muscle in list C. Also, tell the major function of each muscle.

4. Using surface anatomy, palpate each structure in list D.

Injury Assessment

5. Obtain the medical history of an athlete with a suspected thigh injury.

6. Demonstrate how you would observe and identify the clinical signs and symptoms associated with the injuries and conditions in list E.

7. Explain and demonstrate the mechanisms by which each injury in list E occurs. Name the three sports in which each injury is most likely to occur and explain any differences among the injury occurrences and mechanisms in those sports.

8. Demonstrate appropriate sensory, circulatory, and neurological tests for the injuries in list E.

9. Palpate and assess the integrity of the bones and soft tissues associated with each injury in list E.

10. Demonstrate the use of manual muscle testing and other tests as appropriate to assess the flexibility and strength of the muscles associated with each injury in list E.

11. Demonstrate functional and activity-specific tests to determine the integrity of each structure involved in each injury in list E.

Injury Management

12. Explain and demonstrate the appropriate immediate care procedures for each injury in list E. Explain the objectives and criteria for progressing for each step in the procedure.

13. Demonstrate a complete rehabilitation program for each injury in list E. As you proceed, explain the objectives and procedures of each step in the program. Explain the measurement criteria for advancing from one step to another.

Risk Management

14. Using pictures or illustrations, explain the objectives and procedures of prophylactic taping, padding, and bandaging, as appropriate, for the injuries in list E.

15. Demonstrate or explain procedures for preventing each injury in list E.

References

AAOS 1999 (pp. 400-434)

Anderson, Hall, and Martin 2000 (pp. 393-430)

Arnheim and Prentice 2000 (pp. 565-576, 594-599)

Houglum 2001 (pp. 835-903)

Shultz, Houglum, and Perrin 2000 (pp. 269-309)

Starkey and Ryan 2002 (pp. 271-302)

Mastery and Demonstration

Practice and reinforce these competencies by reviewing your class notes and texts, observing peer teachers and certified/licensed professionals perform the skills, discussing the competencies with peer teachers and certified/licensed professionals, practicing alone and with a peer, and then demonstrating proficiency to a peer teacher. Finally, demonstrate your proficiency to an ACI.

Approved by (date and signature)

1. Bones

    Peer _____

    ACI _____

2. Joints

    Peer _____

    ACI _____

3. Muscles

    Peer _____

    ACI _____

4. Other structures

    Peer _____

    ACI _____

5. History

    Peer _____

    ACI _____

6-15. Complete competencies 6-15 for the injuries or conditions in list E:

- Quadriceps contusion

    Peer _____

    ACI _____

- Quadriceps strain

    Peer _____

    ACI _____

- Hamstring strain

  Peer _____

  ACI _____

- Femoral fracture

  Peer _____

  ACI _____

- Myositis ossificans

  Peer _____

  ACI _____

- Patellar tendon rupture

  Peer _____

  ACI _____

Comments

Hip and Pelvic Injury Management

Objective

Develop and demonstrate the skills necessary to properly evaluate, care for, rehabilitate, and prevent hip and pelvic injuries.

Anatomy and Conditions for This Module

A. Bones and Prominent Bony Features

- Ilium
  - Crest
  - Tubercle
  - Anterior inferior spine
  - Anterior superior spine
  - Posterior superior spine
- Pubis
  - Ramus
  - Tubercle
- Ischium
  - Tubercle or tuberosity
- Femur
  - Greater trochanter
  - Lesser trochanter
  - Linea aspera
  - Fovea capitus
- Spine
  - Lumbar vertebrae
  - Sacrum
  - Coccyx

B. Articulations

- Sacroiliac
- Lumbosacral
- Hip
- Pubic symphysis

C. Ligaments

- Inguinal

- Supraspinous
- Interspinous
- Intertransverse
- Longitudinal (posterior and anterior)
- Iliofemoral
- Iliotibial band

D. Muscles

- Gluteus maximus
- Gluteus medius
- Gluteus minimus
- Tensor fasciae latae
- Biceps femoris (long and short heads)
- Semitendinosus
- Semimembranosus
- Iliopsoas
- Psoas major
- Iliacus
- Rectus femoris
- Sartorius
- Gracilis
- Adductor brevis
- Adductor magnus
- Latissimus dorsi
- Paraspinal
- External obliques
- Internal obliques
- Transverse abdominis

E. Other Structures

- Sciatic nerve
- Lateral cutaneous nerve
- Trochanteric bursae
- Iliopsoas bursae
- Male genitalia
- Female genitalia

Ar · · · · · · · · · · Di· ca· · n · subluxation

cial 1 · · · · · · · · · · · · ·gia

· · · ome

· · ·ndrome

· · ·sis—fibular head

· · · must be performed.

· · ·d Assessment of Structural

· · ·te each bone and bony struc-
· · ·lso, tell what differences you
· · ·feel if the bone was fractured.

· · ·the joint line for each articu-
· · ·Then perform active and pas-
· · · tests using both qualitative
· · ·techniques (e.g., tape mea-
· · ·r, and inclinometer). Record
· · ·ests using accepted forms and

· · ·natomy, palpate or draw the
· · ·rse of each ligament in list C.

· · ·natomy, palpate the origin,
· · ·ourse of each muscle in list D.
· · ·jor function of each muscle.

· · ·natomy, palpate each structure

· · ·ical history of an athlete with
· · ·and pelvis injury.

· · ·roper administration and in-
· · ·the special tests in list F.

· · ·w you would observe and iden-
· · ·igns and symptoms associated
· · ·s and conditions in list G.

· · ·nonstrate the mechanisms by
· · ·ry in list G occurs. Name the
· · ·hich each injury is most likely

to occur and explain any differences among the injury occurrences and mechanisms in those sports.

10. Demonstrate appropriate sensory, circulatory, and neurological tests for the injuries in list G.

11. Palpate and assess the integrity of the bones and soft tissues associated with each injury in list G.

12. Perform special tests to assess the integrity of the joints involved in each injury in list G and explain how you would interpret these tests.

13. Demonstrate the use of manual muscle testing and other tests as appropriate to assess the flexibility and strength of the muscles associated with each injury in list G.

14. Demonstrate functional and activity-specific tests to determine the integrity of each structure involved in each injury in list G.

Injury Management

15. Explain and demonstrate the appropriate immediate care procedures for each injury in list G. Explain the objectives and criteria for progressing for each step in the procedure.

16. Demonstrate a complete rehabilitation program for each injury in list G. As you proceed, explain the objectives and procedures of each step in the program. Explain the measurement criteria for advancing from one step to another.

Risk Management

17. Using pictures or illustrations, explain the objectives and procedures of prophylactic taping, padding, and bandaging, as appropriate, for the injuries in list G.

18. Demonstrate or explain procedures for preventing each injury in list G.

References

AAOS 1999 (pp. 400-434)

Anderson, Hall, and Martin 2000 (pp. 393-430)

Arnheim and Prentice 2000 (pp. 576-599)

Houglum 2001 (pp. 907-954)

Magee 1997 (pp. 434-502)

Shultz, Houglum, and Perrin 2000 (pp. 311-348)

Starkey and Ryan 2002 (pp. 272-302)

Mastery and Demonstration

Practice and reinforce these competencies by reviewing your class notes and texts, observing peer teachers and certified/licensed professionals perform the skills, discussing the competencies with peer teachers and certified/licensed professionals, practicing alone and with a peer, and then demonstrating proficiency to a peer teacher. Finally, demonstrate your proficiency to an ACI.

Approved by (date and signature)

1. Bones

Peer _____

ACI _____

2. Joints

Peer _____

ACI _____

3. Ligaments

Peer _____

ACI _____

4. Muscles

Peer _____

ACI _____

5. Other structures

Peer _____

ACI _____

6. History

Peer _____

ACI _____

7. Special Tests

- Leg length discrepancies

Peer _____

ACI _____

- Patrick's/FABER

Peer _____

ACI _____

- Gaenslen's test

  Peer _____

  ACI _____

- Pelvic compression/distraction test

  Peer _____

  ACI _____

- Femoral nerve traction test

  Peer _____

  ACI _____

- Trendelenburg's test

  Peer _____

  ACI _____

- Thomas test

  Peer _____

  ACI _____

- Rectus femoris contracture test

  Peer _____

  ACI _____

- Ober's test

  Peer _____

  ACI _____

- Noble's test

  Peer _____

  ACI _____

- Piriformis test

  Peer _____

  ACI _____

- Straight leg lifting test

  Peer _____

  ACI _____

8-18. Complete competencies 8-18 for the injuries or conditions in list G:

- Snapping hip

  Peer _____

  ACI _____

- Lateral hip pain

  Peer _____

  ACI _____

- Hip retroversion

  Peer _____

  ACI _____

- Hip anteversion

  Peer _____

  ACI _____

- Hip sprain

  Peer _____

  ACI _____

- Contused iliac crest

  Peer _____

  ACI _____

- Dislocated hip

  Peer _____

  ACI _____

- Proximal hamstring strain

  Peer _____

  ACI _____

- Proximal sartorius strain

  Peer _____

  ACI _____

- Hip flexor strain

  Peer _____

  ACI _____

- Hip adductor strain

  Peer _____

  ACI _____

- Gluteal strain

  Peer _____

  ACI _____

- Hernia

  Peer _____

  ACI _____

- Contused genitalia

  Peer _____

  ACI _____

- Spermatic cord torsion

  Peer _____

  ACI _____

- Traumatic hydrocele of the tunica vaginalis

  Peer _____

  ACI _____

- Femur fracture

  Peer _____

  ACI _____

- Pelvic fracture

  Peer _____

  ACI _____

- Trochanteric bursitis

  Peer _____

  ACI _____

- Iliopsoas bursitis

  Peer _____

  ACI _____

- Sacroiliac dysfunction

  Peer _____

  ACI _____

- Legg-Calvé-Perthes disease

  Peer _____

  ACI _____

- Apophysitis

  Peer _____

  ACI _____

- Slipped capital femoral epiphysis

  Peer _____

  ACI _____

- Dislocation or subluxation

  Peer _____

  ACI _____

- Stress fracture

  Peer _____

  ACI _____

- Osteitis pubis

  Peer _____

  ACI _____

- Athletic pubalgia

  Peer _____

  ACI _____

- Bursitis

  Peer _____

  ACI _____

- Piriformis syndrome

  Peer _____

  ACI _____

- Iliotibial band syndrome

  Peer _____

  ACI _____

- Contusion

  Peer _____

  ACI _____

- Tendinitis

  Peer _____

  ACI _____

- Arthritis

  Peer _____

  ACI _____

- Avascular necrosis—fibular head

  Peer _____

  ACI _____

Comments

Thorax and Lumbar Spine Injury Management

Objective

Develop and demonstrate the skills necessary to properly evaluate, care for, rehabilitate, and prevent low back injuries.

Anatomy and Conditions for This Module

A. Bones and Prominent Bony Features

- Ilium
  - Crest
  - Tubercle
  - Anterior inferior spine
  - Anterior superior spine
  - Posterior superior spine
- Pubis
  - Tubercle
- Ischium
  - Tubercle or tuberosity
- Femur
  - Greater trochanter
- Spine
  - Thoracic vertebrae
  - Lumbar vertebrae
  - Spinous processes
  - Sacrum
  - Coccyx

B. Articulations

- Sacroiliac
- Lumbosacral
- Hip
- Thoracic intervertebral
- Lumbar intervertebral
- Costothoracic

C. Ligaments

- Supraspinous
- Interspinous
- Intertransverse
- Longitudinal (posterior and anterior)

D. Muscles

- Rhomboids
- Lower trapezius
- Rectus abdominis
- External oblique
- Internal oblique
- Transverse abdominis
- Gluteus maximus
- Gluteus medius
- Gluteus minimus
- Tensor fasciae latae
- Hamstrings
- Iliopsoas
- Psoas major
- Iliacus
- Paraspinal

E. Other Structures

- Bladder
- Liver
- Spleen
- Kidneys
- Pancreas
- Gall bladder
- Stomach
- Small intestine
- Large intestine

F. Special Tests

- Spinal posture (kyphosis/lordosis)
- Leg length discrepancies
- Valsalva's maneuver + pn
- Straight leg raise test – sciatic nerve
- Well straight leg test – lesion
- Babinski's reflex test
- Oppenheim's gait test
- Kernig's sign – nerve root imp
- Brudzinski's sign test
- Bowstring test
- Hoover's sign test –
- Stork standing test/spondylolisthesis test
- Spring test – spinous process

G. Injuries and Conditions

- Café au lait macules (spots)
- Dislocation or subluxation
- Thoracic sprain/strain
- Lumbar sprain/strain
- Lumbosacral sprain/strain
- Contusion
- Sacroiliac dysfunction
- Intervertebral disc pathology
- Facet syndrome
- Nerve root compression
- Stenosis
- Step deformity
- Sciatica
- Spondylolysis
- Spondylolisthesis
- Spondylitis
- Scoliosis
- Transverse spinous process fracture
- Spina bifida occulta

Competencies

Note: All procedures must be performed.

Anatomical Review and Assessment of Structural Integrity

1. Name and palpate each bone and bony structure in list A. Also, tell what differences you would expect to feel if the bone was fractured.

2. Palpate or draw the joint line for each articulation in list B. Then perform active and passive joint ROM tests using both qualitative and quantitative techniques (e.g., tape measure, goniometer, and inclinometer). Record results of these tests using accepted forms and procedures.

3. Using surface anatomy, palpate or draw the origins and course of each ligament in list C.

4. Using surface anatomy, palpate the origin, insertion, and course of each muscle in list D. Also, tell the major function of each muscle.

5. Using surface anatomy, palpate each structure in list E.

Injury Assessment

6. Obtain the medical history of an athlete with a suspected thoracic or lumbar spine injury.

7. Demonstrate proper administration and interpretation of the special tests in list F.

8. Demonstrate how you would observe and identify the clinical signs and symptoms associated with the injuries and conditions in list G.

9. Explain and demonstrate the mechanisms by which each injury in list G occurs. Name the three sports in which each injury is most likely to occur and explain any differences among the injury occurrences and mechanisms in those sports.

10. Demonstrate appropriate sensory, circulatory, and neurological tests for the injuries in list G.

11. Palpate and assess the integrity of the bones and soft tissues associated with each injury in list G.

12. Perform special tests to assess the integrity of the joints involved in each injury in list G and explain how you would interpret these tests.

13. Demonstrate the use of manual muscle testing and other tests as appropriate to assess the flexibility and strength of the muscles associated with each injury in list G.

14. Demonstrate functional and activity-specific tests to determine the integrity of each structure involved in each injury in list G

Injury Management

15. Explain and demonstrate the appropriate immediate care procedures for each injury in list G. Explain the objectives and criteria for progressing for each step in the procedure.

16. Demonstrate a complete rehabilitation program for each injury in list G. As you proceed, explain the objectives and procedures of each step in the program. Explain the measurement criteria for advancing from one step to another.

Risk Management

17. Using pictures or illustrations, explain the objectives and procedures of prophylactic taping, padding, and bandaging, as appropriate, for the injuries in list G.

18. Demonstrate or explain procedures for preventing each injury in list G.

References

AAOS 1999 (pp. 369-398)

Anderson, Hall, and Martin 2000 (pp. 535-583)

Arnheim and Prentice 2000 (pp. 634-683)

Houglum 2001 (pp. 497-563)

Magee 1997 (pp. 331-428)

Shultz, Houglum, and Perrin 2000 (pp. 199-227)

Starkey and Ryan 2002 (pp. 319-368)

Mastery and Demonstration

Practice and reinforce these competencies by reviewing your class notes and texts, observing peer teachers and certified/licensed professionals perform the skills, discussing the competencies with peer teachers and certified/licensed professionals, practicing alone and with a peer, and then demonstrating proficiency to a peer teacher. Finally, demonstrate your proficiency to an ACI.

Approved by (date and signature)

1. Bones

Peer_____

ACI_____

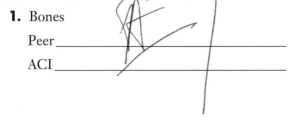

2. Joints

Peer_____

ACI_____

3. Ligaments

Peer_____

ACI_____

4. Muscles

Peer_____

ACI_____

5. Other structures

Peer_____

ACI_____

6. History

Peer_____

ACI_____

7. Special Tests

- Spinal posture

  Peer_____

  ACI_____

- Leg length discrepancies

  Peer_____

  ACI_____

- Valsalva's maneuver

  Peer_____

  ACI_____

- Straight leg raise test

  Peer_____

  ACI_____

- Well straight leg test

  Peer_____

  ACI_____

- Babinski's reflex test

  Peer_____

  ACI_____

- Oppenheim's gait test

  Peer _____

  ACI _____

- Kernig's sign

  Peer _____

  ACI _____

- Brudzinski's sign test

  Peer _____

  ACI _____

- Bowstring test

  Peer _____

  ACI _____

- Hoover's sign test

  Peer _____

  ACI _____

- Stork standing test/spondylolisthesis test

  Peer _____

  ACI _____

- Spring test

  Peer _____

  ACI _____

8-18. Complete competencies 8-18 for the injuries or conditions in list G:

- Café au lait macules

  Peer _____

  ACI _____

- Dislocation or subluxation

  Peer _____

  ACI _____

- Thoracic sprain/strain

  Peer _____

  ACI _____

- Lumbar sprain/strain

  Peer _____

  ACI _____

- Lumbosacral sprain/strain

  Peer _____

  ACI _____

- Contusion

  Peer _____

  ACI _____

- Sacroiliac dysfunction

  Peer _____

  ACI _____

- Disc pathology

  Peer _____

  ACI _____

- Facet syndrome

  Peer _____

  ACI _____

- Nerve root compression

  Peer _____

  ACI _____

- Stenosis

  Peer _____

  ACI _____

- Step deformity

  Peer _____

  ACI _____

- Sciatica

  Peer _____

  ACI _____

- Spondylolysis

  Peer _____

  ACI _____

- Spondylolisthesis

  Peer _____

  ACI _____

- Spondylitis

  Peer _____

  ACI _____

- Scoliosis

  Peer _____

  ACI _____

- Transverse spinous process fracture

  Peer _____

  ACI _____

- Spina bifida occulta

  Peer _____

  ACI _____

Comments

Thorax and Abdominal Injury Management

Objective

Develop and demonstrate the skills necessary to properly evaluate, care for, rehabilitate, and prevent thorax and abdominal injuries.

Anatomy and Conditions for This Module

A. Bones and Prominent Bony Features

- Ilium
  - Crest
  - Tubercle
  - Anterior inferior spine
  - Anterior superior spine
  - Posterior superior spine
- Spine
  - Thoracic vertebrae
  - Lumbar vertebrae
  - Spinous processes
- Rib cage
  - Ribs
  - Floating ribs
  - Costal cartilage
- Sternum
  - Manubrium
  - Body
  - Xiphoid process

B. Articulations

- Sternoclavicular
- Costosternal
- Costovertebral
- Costochondral

C. Muscles

- Rectus abdominis
- Obliques
- Transverse abdominis
- Latissimus dorsi
- Erector spinae
- Quadratus lumborum
- Intercostals
- Diaphragm

D. Other Structures

- Phrenic nerve
- Heart UL
- Lungs UL&R
- Pancreas
- Liver UR
- Spleen
- Kidneys
- Stomach
- Intestine
- Gallbladder
- Urinary bladder

E. Injuries and Conditions

- Abdominal muscular strain
- Rectus abdominis contusion
- Spleen rupture
- Kidney contusion
- Stitch in the side
- Wind knocked out
- SC separation
- Sternal fracture
- Rib fracture
- Rib contusion
- Costochondral dislocation
- Pneumothorax
- Hemothorax

Competencies

Note: All procedures must be performed.

Anatomical Review and Assessment of Structural Integrity

1. Name and palpate each bone and bony structures in list A. Also, tell what differences you would expect to feel if the bone was fractured.

2. Palpate or draw the joint line for each articulation in list B. Then perform active and passive joint ROM tests using both qualitative and quantitative techniques (e.g., tape measure, goniometer, and inclinometer). Record results of these tests using accepted forms and procedures.

3. Using surface anatomy, palpate the origin, insertion, and course of each muscle in list C. Also, tell the major function of each muscle.

4. Using surface anatomy, palpate each structure in list D.

Injury Assessment

5. Obtain the medical history of an athlete with a suspected thorax or abdominal injury.

6. Demonstrate how you would observe and identify the clinical signs and symptoms associated with the injuries and conditions in list E.

7. Explain and demonstrate the mechanisms by which each injury in list E occurs. Name the three sports in which each injury is most likely to occur and explain any differences among the injury occurrences and mechanisms in those sports.

8. Demonstrate appropriate sensory, circulatory, and neurological tests for the injuries in list E.

9. Palpate and assess the integrity of the bones and soft tissues associated with each injury in list E.

10. Perform special tests to assess the integrity of the joints involved in each injury in list E and explain how you would interpret these tests.

11. Demonstrate the use of manual muscle testing and other tests as appropriate to assess the flexibility and strength of the muscles associated with each injury in list E.

12. Demonstrate functional and activity-specific tests to determine the integrity of each structure involved in each injury in list E.

Injury Management

13. Explain and demonstrate the appropriate immediate care procedures for each injury in list E. Explain the objectives and criteria for progressing for each step in the procedure.

14. Demonstrate a complete rehabilitation program for each injury in list E. As you proceed, explain the objectives and procedures of each step in the program. Explain the measurement criteria for advancing from one step to another.

Risk Management

15. Using pictures or illustrations, explain the objectives and procedures of prophylactic taping, padding, and bandaging, as appropriate, for the injuries in list E.

16. Demonstrate or explain procedures for preventing each injury in list E.

References

AAOS 1999 (pp. 356-377)

Anderson, Hall, and Martin 2000 (pp. 251-279)

Arnheim and Prentice 2000 (pp. 751-783)

Houglum 2001 (pp. 456-467, 507-538)

Shultz, Houglum, and Perrin 2000 (pp. 381-405)

Starkey and Ryan 2002 (pp. 395-423)

Mastery and Demonstration

Practice and reinforce these competencies by reviewing your class notes and texts, observing peer teachers and certified/licensed professionals perform the skills, discussing the competencies with peer teachers and certified/licensed professionals, practicing alone and with a peer, and then demonstrating proficiency to a peer teacher. Finally, demonstrate your proficiency to an ACI.

Approved by (date and signature)

1. Bones

Peer _Dana C._____

ACI_____

Module J8—Thorax and Abdominal Injury Management (continued)

2. Joints

Peer _____

ACI _____

3. Muscles

Peer _____

ACI _____

4. Other structures

Peer _____

ACI _____

5. History

Peer _____

ACI _____

6-16. Complete competencies 6-16 for the injuries or conditions in list E:

- Abdominal strain

  Peer _____

  ACI _____

- Rectus abdominis contusion

  Peer _____

  ACI _____

- Spleen rupture

  Peer _____

  ACI _____

- Kidney contusion

  Peer _____

  ACI _____

- Stitch in side

  Peer _____

  ACI _____

- Wind knocked out

  Peer _____

  ACI _____

- SC separation

  Peer _____

  ACI _____

- Sternal fracture

  Peer _____

  ACI _____

- Rib fracture

  Peer _____

  ACI _____

- Rib contusion

  Peer _____

  ACI _____

- Costochondral dislocation

  Peer _____

  ACI _____

- Pneumothorax

  Peer _____

  ACI _____

- Hemothorax

  Peer _____

  ACI _____

Comments

LEVEL 3   Module J9
Specific Injury Management

Shoulder Injury Management

Objective

Develop and demonstrate the skills necessary to properly evaluate, care for, rehabilitate, and prevent shoulder injuries.

Anatomy and Conditions for This Module

A. Bones and Prominent Bony Features

- Ribs
- Sternum
  - Manubrium
  - Body
- Clavicle
- Scapula
  - Suprapatellar fossa
  - Spine
  - Infrapatellar fossa
  - Acromion process
  - Coracoid process
  - Medial border
  - Lateral border
  - Inferior angle
- Humerus
  - Greater trochanter
  - Lesser trochanter
  - Bicipital groove

B. Articulations

- Glenohumeral
- Acromioclavicular
- Coracoclaviular
- Sternoclavicular
- Scapulothoracic

C. Ligaments

- Glenohumeral
  - Anterior
  - Middle
  - Posterior
- Acromioclavicular
- Coracoclavicular
- Coracoacromial
- Sternoclavicular

D. Muscles

1. Biceps (both heads)
2. Triceps (all three heads)
3. Deltoid (all three portions)
4. Pectoralis major
5. Pectoralis minor
6. Teres major
7. Teres minor
8. Latissimus dorsi
9. Supraspinatus
10. Infraspinatus
11. Subscapularis
12. Trapezius
13. Rhomboids
14. Levator scapulae
15. Serratus anterior
16. Subclavius

E. Other Structures

- Subacromial bursa
- Subdeltoid bursa
- Brachial plexus
- Axillary nerve

F. Special Tests

- Symmetry
- Efficiency of movement

- Scapulohumeral rhythm
- Anterior drawer test
- Posterior drawer test
- Relocation test
- Apprehension test
- Clunk test
- Sulcus sign
- Shear test
- Compression test
- Speed's test
- Drop arm test
- Empty can test
- Impingement test
- Hawkins-Kennedy impingement test
- Neer's impingement test
- Pectoralis major contracture test
- Yergason's test
- Ludington's test
- Adson's maneuver
- Allen's test
- Military brace position

G. Injuries and Conditions

1. Fracture
2. Nerve injury
3. Step deformity
4. Scapular winging
5. Sternoclavicular sprain/dislocation
6. Clavicular fracture
7. Acromioclavicular instability
8. Glenohumeral instability
9. Recurrent glenohumeral dislocation
10. Subacromial impingement
11. Rotator cuff strain
12. Subacromial bursitis
13. Tenosynovitis and tendinitis
14. Bicipital subluxation
15. Thoracic outlet syndrome
16. Epiphyseal fracture
17. Throwing injuries
18. Sprengel's deformity

Competencies

Note: All procedures must be performed.

Anatomical Review and Assessment of Structural Integrity

1. Name and palpate each bone and bony structures in list A. Also, tell what differences you would expect to feel if the bone was fractured.

2. Palpate or draw the joint line for each articulation in list B. Then perform active and passive joint ROM tests using both qualitative and quantitative techniques (e.g., tape measure, goniometer, and inclinometer). Record results of these tests using accepted forms and procedures.

3. Using surface anatomy, palpate or draw the origins and course of each ligament in list C.

4. Using surface anatomy, palpate the origin, insertion, and course of each muscle in list D. Also, tell the major function of each muscle.

5. Using surface anatomy, palpate each structure in list E.

Injury Assessment

6. Obtain the medical history of an athlete with a suspected shoulder injury.

7. Demonstrate proper administration and interpretation of the special tests in list F.

8. Demonstrate how you would observe and identify the clinical signs and symptoms associated with the injuries and conditions in list G.

9. Explain and demonstrate the mechanisms by which each injury in list G occur. Name the three sports in which each injury is most likely to occur and explain any differences among the injury occurrences and mechanisms in those sports.

10. Demonstrate appropriate sensory, circulatory, and neurological tests for the injuries in list G.

11. Palpate and assess the integrity of the bones and soft tissues associated with each injury in list G.

12. Perform special tests to assess the integrity of the joints involved in each injury in list G and explain how you would interpret these tests.

13. Demonstrate the use of manual muscle testing and other tests as appropriate to assess the flexibility and strength of the muscles associated with each injury in list G.

14. Demonstrate functional and activity-specific tests to determine the integrity of each structure involved in each injury in list G.

Injury Management

15. Explain and demonstrate the appropriate immediate care procedures for each injury in list G. Explain the objectives and criteria for progressing for each step in the procedure.

16. Demonstrate a complete rehabilitation program for each injury in list G. As you proceed, explain the objectives and procedures of each step in the program. Explain the measurement criteria for advancing from one step to another.

Risk Management

17. Using pictures or illustrations, explain the objectives and procedures of prophylactic taping, padding, and bandaging, as appropriate, for the injuries in list G.

18. Demonstrate or explain procedures for preventing each injury in list G.

References

AAOS 1991 (pp. 220-291)

Anderson, Hall, and Martin 2000 (pp. 282-325)

Arnheim and Prentice 2000 (pp. 600-644)

Houglum 2001 (pp. 565-655)

Magee 1997 (pp. 170-240)

Shultz, Houglum, and Perrin 2000 (pp. 84-125)

Starkey and Ryan 2002 (pp. 424-488)

Mastery and Demonstration

Practice and reinforce these competencies by reviewing your class notes and texts, observing peer teachers and certified/licensed professionals perform the skills, discussing the competencies with peer teachers and certified/licensed professionals, practicing alone and with a peer, and then demonstrating proficiency to a peer teacher. Finally, demonstrate your proficiency to an ACI.

Approved by (date and signature)

1. Bones

Peer _____

ACI _____

2. Joints

Peer _____

ACI _____

3. Ligaments

Peer _____

ACI _____

4. Muscles

Peer _____

ACI _____

5. Other structures

Peer _____

ACI _____

6. History

Peer _____

ACI _____

7. Special Tests

- Symmetry

  Peer _____

  ACI _____

- Efficiency of movement

  Peer _____

  ACI _____

- Scapulohumeral rhythm

  Peer _____

  ACI _____

- Anterior drawer test

  Peer _____

  ACI _____

- Posterior drawer test

  Peer _____

  ACI _____

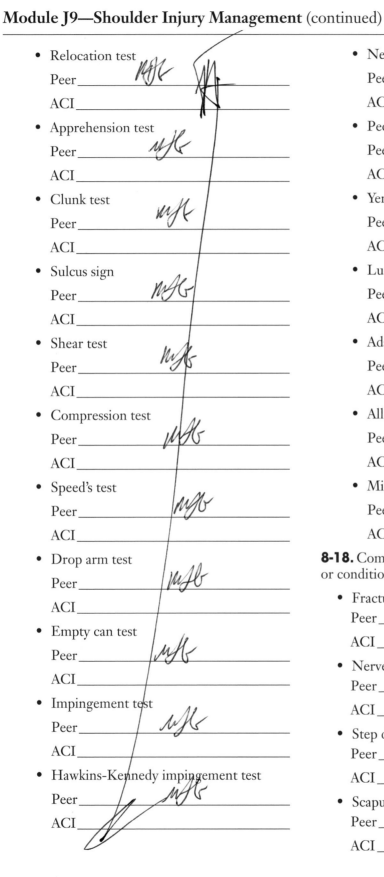

- Relocation test
  Peer
  ACI
- Apprehension test
  Peer
  ACI
- Clunk test
  Peer
  ACI
- Sulcus sign
  Peer
  ACI
- Shear test
  Peer
  ACI
- Compression test
  Peer
  ACI
- Speed's test
  Peer
  ACI
- Drop arm test
  Peer
  ACI
- Empty can test
  Peer
  ACI
- Impingement test
  Peer
  ACI
- Hawkins-Kennedy impingement test
  Peer
  ACI

- Neer's impingement test
  Peer
  ACI
- Pectoralis major contracture test
  Peer
  ACI
- Yergason's test
  Peer
  ACI
- Ludington's test
  Peer
  ACI
- Adson's maneuver
  Peer
  ACI
- Allen's test
  Peer
  ACI
- Military brace position
  Peer
  ACI

8-18. Complete competencies 8-18 for the injuries or conditions in list G:

- Fracture
  Peer
  ACI
- Nerve injury
  Peer
  ACI
- Step deformity
  Peer
  ACI
- Scapular winging
  Peer
  ACI

Module J9—Shoulder Injury Management (continued)

- Sternoclavicular sprain/dislocation

  Peer

  ACI

- Clavicular fracture

  Peer

  ACI

- Acromioclavicular instability

  Peer

  ACI

- Glenohumeral instability

  Peer

  ACI

- Recurrent glenohumeral dislocation

  Peer

  ACI

- Subacromial impingement

  Peer

  ACI

- Rotator cuff strain

  Peer

  ACI

- Subacromial bursitis

  Peer

  ACI

- Tenosynovitis and tendinitis

  Peer

  ACI

- Bicipital subluxation

  Peer

  ACI

- Thoracic outlet syndrome

  Peer

  ACI

- Epiphyseal fracture

  Peer

  ACI

- Throwing injuries

  Peer

  ACI

- Sprengel's deformity

  Peer

  ACI

Comments

Specific Injury Management

Arm and Elbow Injury Management

Objective

Develop and demonstrate the skills necessary to properly evaluate, care for, rehabilitate, and prevent arm and elbow injuries.

Anatomy and Conditions for This Module

A. Bones and Prominent Bony Features

- Humerus
  - Greater trochanter
  - Lesser trochanter
  - Bicipital groove
  - Capitulum
  - Olecranon fossa
  - Trochlea
- Ulna
  - Olecranon process
  - Coronoid process
  - Trochlea notch
  - Radial notch
  - Interosseous border
- Radius
  - Head
  - Interosseous border
  - Ulnar notch

B. Articulations

- Radiohumeral
- Ulnahumeral
- Proximal radioulnar

C. Ligaments

- Annular
- Ulnar collateral
- Radial collateral
- Interosseous

D. Muscles

- Biceps (both heads)
- Triceps (all three heads)
- Coracobrachialis
- Brachialis
- Brachioradialis
- Anconeus
- Pronator teres
- Pronator quadratus
- Flexor carpi radialis
- Flexor carpi ulnaris
- Extensor digitorum
- Supinator

E. Other Structures

- Median nerve
- Radial nerve
- Ulnar nerve
- Radial artery
- Olecranon bursa
- Radiohumeral bursa

F. Special Tests

- Symmetry
- Carrying angle (cubital valgus and varus)
- Efficiency of movement
- Tenosynovitis and tendinitis
- Muscle atrophy
- Valgus stress test
- Varus stress test
- Lateral epicondylitis inflammation
- Medial epicondylitis inflammation
- Tinel's sign
- Pinch grip test

G. Injuries and Conditions

- Bicipital strain
- Humeral fracture
- Epiphyseal fracture
- Humeral contusion
- Humeral exostoses
- Supracondylar fracture
- Olecranon bursitis
- Medial elbow strain
- Medial collateral ligament sprain
- Elbow hyperextension
- Elbow dislocation
- Elbow fracture
- Radial nerve injury
- Throwing injury
- Medial epicondylitis
- Lateral epicondylitis
- Forearm contusion
- Radial head fracture
- Forearm splint
- Dislocation or subluxation
- Pronator teres syndrome
- Nerve injury
- Bursitis
- Osteochondritis dissecans

Competencies

Note: All procedures must be performed.

Anatomical Review and Assessment of Structural Integrity

1. Name and palpate each bone and bony structure in list A. Also, tell what differences you would expect to feel if the bone was fractured.

2. Palpate or draw the joint line for each articulation in list B. Then perform active and passive joint ROM tests using both qualitative and quantitative techniques (e.g., tape measure, goniometer, and inclinometer). Record results of these tests using accepted forms and procedures.

3. Using surface anatomy, palpate or draw the origins and course of each ligament in list C.

4. Using surface anatomy, palpate the origin, insertion, and course of each muscle in list D. Also, tell the major function of each muscle.

5. Using surface anatomy, palpate each structure in list E.

Injury Assessment

6. Obtain the medical history of an athlete with a suspected arm or elbow injury.

7. Demonstrate proper administration and interpretation of the special tests in list F.

8. Demonstrate how you would observe and identify the clinical signs and symptoms associated with the injuries and conditions in list G.

9. Explain and demonstrate the mechanisms by which each injury in list G occurs. Name the three sports in which each injury is most likely to occur and explain any differences among the injury occurrences and mechanisms in those sports.

10. Demonstrate appropriate sensory, circulatory, and neurological tests for the injuries in list G.

11. Palpate and assess the integrity of the bones and soft tissues associated with each injury in list G.

12. Perform special tests to assess the integrity of the joints involved in each injury in list G and explain how you would interpret these tests.

13. Demonstrate the use of manual muscle testing and other tests as appropriate to assess the flexibility and strength of the muscles associated with each injury in list G.

14. Demonstrate functional and activity-specific tests to determine the integrity of each structure involved in each injury in list G.

Injury Management

15. Explain and demonstrate the appropriate immediate care procedures for each injury in list G. Explain the objectives and criteria for progressing for each step in the procedure.

16. Demonstrate a complete rehabilitation program for each injury in list G. As you proceed, explain the objectives and procedures of each step in the program. Explain the measurement criteria for advancing from one step to another.

Risk Management

17. Using pictures or illustrations, explain the objectives and procedures of prophylactic taping, padding, and bandaging, as appropriate, for the injuries in list G.

18. Demonstrate or explain procedures for preventing each injury in list G.

References

AAOS 1999 (pp. 294-334)

Anderson, Hall, and Martin 2000 (pp. 326-355)

Arnheim and Prentice 2000 (pp. 645-670)

Houglum 2001 (pp. 657-699)

Magee 1997 (pp. 247-272)

Shultz, Houglum, and Perrin 2000 (pp. 127-160)

Starkey and Ryan 2002 (pp. 424-517)

Mastery and Demonstration

Practice and reinforce these competencies by reviewing your class notes and texts, observing peer teachers and certified/licensed professionals perform the skills, discussing the competencies with peer teachers and certified/licensed professionals, practicing alone and with a peer, and then demonstrating proficiency to a peer teacher. Finally, demonstrate your proficiency to an ACI.

Approved by (date and signature)

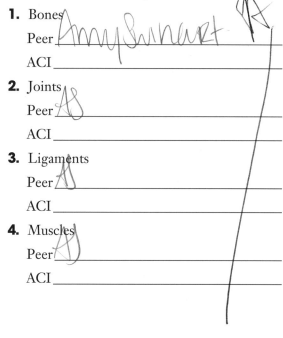

1. Bones

Peer _____

ACI _____

2. Joints

Peer _____

ACI _____

3. Ligaments

Peer _____

ACI _____

4. Muscles

Peer _____

ACI _____

5. Other structures

Peer _____

ACI _____

6. History

Peer _____

ACI _____

7. Special Tests

- Symmetry

  Peer _____

  ACI _____

- Carrying angle

  Peer _____

  ACI _____

- Efficiency of movement

  Peer _____

  ACI _____

- Tenosynovitis and tendinitis

  Peer _____

  ACI _____

- Muscle atrophy

  Peer _____

  ACI _____

- Valgus stress test

  Peer _____

  ACI _____

- Varus stress test

  Peer _____

  ACI _____

- Lateral epicondylitis inflammation

  Peer _____

  ACI _____

- Medial epicondylitis inflammation

  Peer _____

  ACI _____

- Tinel's sign
  Peer
  ACI

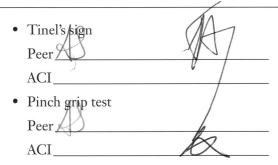

- Pinch grip test
  Peer
  ACI

8-18. Complete competencies 8-18 for the injuries or conditions in list G:

- Bicipital strain
  Peer
  ACI

- Humeral fracture
  Peer
  ACI

- Epiphyseal fracture
  Peer
  ACI

- Humeral contusion
  Peer
  ACI

- Humeral exostoses
  Peer
  ACI

- Supracondylar fracture
  Peer
  ACI

- Olecranon bursitis
  Peer
  ACI

- Medial elbow strain
  Peer
  ACI

- Medial collateral ligament sprain
  Peer
  ACI

- Elbow hyperextension
  Peer
  ACI

- Elbow dislocation
  Peer
  ACI

- Elbow fracture
  Peer
  ACI

- Radial nerve injury
  Peer
  ACI

- Throwing injury
  Peer
  ACI

- Medial epicondylitis
  Peer
  ACI

- Lateral epicondylitis
  Peer
  ACI

- Forearm contusion
  Peer
  ACI

- Radial head fracture
  Peer
  ACI

- Forearm splint
  Peer
  ACI

- Dislocation or subluxation
  Peer
  ACI

- Pronator teres syndrome
  Peer
  ACI

- Nerve injury

  Peer _____

  ACI _____

- Bursitis

  Peer _____

  ACI _____

- Osteochondritis dissecans

  Peer _____

  ACI _____

Comments

Wrist and Hand Injury Management

Objective

Develop and demonstrate the skills necessary to properly evaluate, care for, rehabilitate, and prevent wrist and hand injuries.

Anatomy and Conditions for This Module

A. Bones and Prominent Bony Features

- Ulna
  - Styloid process
- Radius
  - Styloid process
- Pisiform
- Triquetrum
- Lunate
- Scaphoid
- Hamate
- Capitate
- Trapezoid
- Trapezium
- Metacarpals
- Phalanges
  - Proximal
  - Middle
  - Distal

B. Articulations

- Distal radioulnar
- Radiocarpal
- Ulnocarpal
- Midcarpal
- Carpal-metacarpal
- Proximal interphalangeal
- Distal interphalangeal

C. Ligaments

- Flexor retinaculum

- Ulnar collateral
- Radial collateral
- PIP
- DIP
- Palmar
- Deep transverse
- Volar plate

D. Muscles

- Palmaris longus
- Extensor pollicis longus
- Flexor carpi radialis
- Flexor carpi ulnaris
- Brachioradialis
- Extensor carpi radialis
- Extensor carpi ulnaris
- Extensor digitorum
- Lumbricles
- Palmer interossei
- Dorsal interossei

E. Other Structures

- Medial nerve
- Radial nerve
- Ulnar nerve
- Radial pulse
- Thenar eminence
- Hypothenar eminence

F. Special Tests

- Finkelstein's test
- Valgus stress test
- Varus stress test
- Glide test
- Tinel's sign
- Phalen's test

G. Injuries and Conditions

1. • Colles' fracture
2. • Scaphoid fracture
3. • Lunate dislocation
4. • Hamate fracture
5. • Bennett's fracture
6. • Carpal fracture (boxer's fracture)
7. • Radioulnar sprain
8. • Wrist ganglion
9. • Carpal sprain
10. • Carpal tunnel syndrome
11. • Hand contusion
12. • Dupuytren's contracture
13. • Ganglion
14. • Bishop's or benediction deformity
15. • Ape hand
16. • Claw fingers
17. • Drop-wrist deformity
18. • Volkmann's contracture
19. • Metacarpal fracture
20. • Phalangeal fracture
21. • Thumb ulnocollateral ligament sprain
22. • PIP sprain
23. • Flexor tendon avulsion (jersey finger)
24. • Extensor tendon avulsion (mallet finger)
25. • Extensor tendon rupture (boutonniere deformity)
26. • Volar plate rupture (pseudo-boutonniere deformity)
27. • Interphalangeal dislocations
28. • Subungual hematoma
29. • Clubbed nails
30. • Spoon-shaped nails
31. • Swan neck deformity
32. • Trigger finger

Competencies

Note: All procedures must be performed.

Anatomical Review and Assessment of Structural Integrity

1. Name and palpate each bone and bony structure in list A. Also, tell what differences you would expect to feel if the bone was fractured.

2. Palpate or draw the joint line for each articulation in list B. Then perform active and passive joint ROM tests using both qualitative and quantitative techniques (e.g., tape measure, goniometer, and inclinometer). Record results of these tests using accepted forms and procedures.

3. Using surface anatomy, palpate or draw the origins and course of each ligament in list C.

4. Using surface anatomy, palpate the origin, insertion, and course of each muscle in list D. Also, tell the major function of each muscle.

5. Using surface anatomy, palpate each structure in list E.

Injury Assessment

6. Obtain the medical history of an athlete with a suspected wrist or hand injury.

7. Demonstrate proper administration and interpretation of the special tests in list F.

8. Demonstrate how you would observe and identify the clinical signs and symptoms associated with the injuries and conditions in list G.

9. Explain and demonstrate the mechanisms by which each injury in list G occurs. Name the three sports in which each injury is most likely to occur and explain any differences among the injury occurrences and mechanisms in those sports.

10. Demonstrate appropriate sensory, circulatory, and neurological tests for the injuries in list G.

11. Palpate and assess the integrity of the bones and soft tissues associated with each injury in list G.

12. Perform special tests to assess the integrity of the joints involved in each injury in list G and explain how you would interpret these tests.

13. Demonstrate the use of manual muscle testing and other tests as appropriate to assess the flexibility and strength of the muscles associated with each injury in list G.

14. Demonstrate functional and activity-specific tests to determine the integrity of each structure involved in each injury in list G.

Injury Management

15. Explain and demonstrate the appropriate immediate care procedures for each injury in list G. Explain the objectives and criteria for progressing for each step in the procedure.

16. Demonstrate a complete rehabilitation program for each injury in list G. As you proceed, explain the objectives and procedures of each step in the program. Explain the measurement criteria for advancing from one step to another.

Risk Management

17. Using pictures or illustrations, explain the objectives and procedures of prophylactic taping, padding, and bandaging, as appropriate, for the injuries in list G.

18. Demonstrate or explain procedures for preventing each injury in list G.

References

AAOS 1999 (pp. 336-353)

Anderson, Hall, and Martin 2000 (pp. 356-389)

Arnheim and Prentice 2000 (pp. 670-694)

Houglum 2001 (pp. 657-699)

Magee 1997 (pp. 275-327)

Shultz, Houglum, and Perrin 2000 (pp. 162-197)

Starkey and Ryan 2002 (pp. 519-565)

Mastery and Demonstration

Practice and reinforce these competencies by reviewing your class notes and texts, observing peer teachers and certified/licensed professionals perform the skills, discussing the competencies with peer teachers and certified/licensed professionals, practicing alone and with a peer, and then demonstrating proficiency to a peer teacher. Finally, demonstrate your proficiency to an ACI.

Approved by (date and signature)

1. Bones

Peer 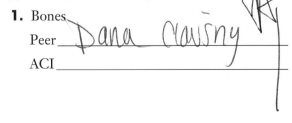 _Dana Craisny_

ACI _____

2. Joints

Peer __ _DC_ __

ACI _____

3. Ligaments

Peer __ _DC_ __

ACI _____

4. Muscles

Peer __ _DC_ __

ACI _____

5. Other structures

Peer __ _DC_ __

ACI _____

6. History

Peer __ _DC_ __

ACI _____

7. Special Tests

• Finkelstein's test

Peer __ _DC_ __

ACI _____

• Valgus stress test

Peer __ _DC_ __

ACI _____

• Varus stress test

Peer __ _DC_ __

ACI _____

• Glide test

Peer __ _DC_ __

ACI _____

• Tinel's sign

Peer __ _DC_ __

ACI _____

• Phalen's test

Peer __ _DC_ __

ACI _____

8-18. Complete competencies 8-18 for the injuries or conditions in list G:

- Colles' fracture
  Peer _DC_____
  ACI_____

- Scaphoid fracture
  Peer_____
  ACI_____

- Lunate dislocation
  Peer_____
  ACI_____

- Hamate fracture
  Peer_____
  ACI_____

- Bennett's fracture
  Peer_____
  ACI_____

- Carpal fracture
  Peer_____
  ACI_____

- Radioulnar sprain
  Peer_____
  ACI_____

- Wrist ganglion
  Peer_____
  ACI_____

- Carpal sprain
  Peer_____
  ACI_____

- Carpal tunnel syndrome
  Peer_____
  ACI_____

- Hand contusion
  Peer_____
  ACI_____

- Dupuytren's contracture
  Peer _DC_____
  ACI_____

- Ganglion
  Peer_____
  ACI_____

- Bishop's deformity
  Peer_____
  ACI_____

- Ape hand
  Peer_____
  ACI_____

- Claw fingers
  Peer_____
  ACI_____

- Drop-wrist deformity
  Peer_____
  ACI_____

- Volkmann's contracture
  Peer_____
  ACI_____

- Metacarpal fracture
  Peer_____
  ACI_____

- Phalangeal fracture
  Peer_____
  ACI_____

- Thumb ulnocollateral
  Peer_____
  ACI_____

- PIP sprain
  Peer_____
  ACI_____

- Flexor tendon avulsion
  Peer_____
  ACI_____

- Extensor tendon avulsion

  Peer _DC_____

  ACI _____

- Extensor tendon rupture

  Peer _____

  ACI _____

- Volar plate rupture

  Peer _____

  ACI _____

- Interphalangeal dislocations

  Peer _____

  ACI _____

- Subungual hematoma

  Peer _____

  ACI _____

- Clubbed nails

  Peer _____

  ACI _____

- Spoon-shaped nails

  Peer _____

  ACI _____

- Swan neck deformity

  Peer _____

  ACI _____

- Trigger finger

  Peer _____

  ACI _____

Comments

12/6/10   5/5

Cervical Spine Injury Management

Objective

Develop and demonstrate the skills necessary to properly evaluate, care for, rehabilitate, and prevent cervical spine injuries.

Anatomy and Conditions for This Module

A. Bones and Prominent Bony Features

- Cervical vertebrae
  - Spinous processes
  - Transverse processes
- Atlas axis *c1*
- Clavicle
- First rib

B. Articulations

- Cervical intervertebral articulation

C. Ligaments

- Nuchal
- Ligamentum flavum *connects vertebrae*
- Ligamentum nuchae

D. Muscles

- Sternocleidomastoid
- Scalene (three portions)
- Trapezius
- Posterior vertebral

E. Other Structures

- Brachial plexus
- Myotomes *motor*
- Dermatomes *sensory*
- Cervical plexus *c1-c5*
- Vertebral artery

F. Special Tests

- Valsalva's maneuver
- Distraction/compression
- Spurling's test
- Shoulder depression
- Vertebral artery test
- Brachial tension test
- Tinel's sign
- Upper extremity neurological evaluation

G. Injuries and Conditions

- Cervical dislocation
- Cervical subluxation
- Cervical sprain
- Cervical strain
- Neck contusion
- Neck burner
- Neck muscle atrophy
- Vertebral fracture
- Faulty head and neck posture
- Intervertebral disc herniation
- Nerve root compression or stretch
- Spinal cord ischemia
- Torticollis
- Brachial plexus neuropathy
- Neurovascular dysfunction
- Vertebral artery occlusion

Competencies

Note: All procedures must be performed.

Anatomical Review and Assessment of Structural Integrity

1. Name and palpate each bone and bony structure in list A. Also, tell what differences you would expect to feel if the bone was fractured.

2. Palpate or draw the joint line for each articulation in list B. Then perform active and passive joint ROM tests using both qualitative and quantitative techniques (e.g., tape measure, goniometer, and inclinometer). Record

results of these tests using accepted forms and procedures.

3. Using surface anatomy, palpate or draw the origins and course of each ligament in list C.

4. Using surface anatomy, palpate the origin, insertion, and course of each muscle in list D. Also, tell the major function of each muscle.

5. Using surface anatomy, palpate each structure in list E.

Injury Assessment

6. Obtain the medical history of an athlete with a suspected cervical spine injury.

7. Demonstrate proper administration and interpretation of the special tests in list F.

8. Demonstrate how you would observe and identify the clinical signs and symptoms associated with the injuries and conditions in list G.

9. Explain and demonstrate the mechanisms by which each injury in list G occurs. Name the three sports in which each injury is most likely to occur and explain any differences among the injury occurrences and mechanisms in those sports.

10. Demonstrate appropriate sensory, circulatory, and neurological tests for the injuries in list G.

11. Palpate and assess the integrity of the bones and soft tissues associated with each injury in list G.

12. Perform special tests to assess the integrity of the joints involved in each injury in list G and explain how you would interpret these tests.

13. Demonstrate the use of manual muscle testing and other tests as appropriate to assess the flexibility and strength of the muscles associated with each injury in list G.

14. Demonstrate functional and activity-specific tests to determine the integrity of each structure involved in each injury in list G.

Injury Management

15. Explain and demonstrate the appropriate immediate care procedures for each injury in list G. Explain the objectives and criteria for progressing for each step in the procedure.

16. Demonstrate a complete rehabilitation program for each injury in list G. As you proceed, explain the objectives and procedures of each step in the program. Explain the measurement criteria for advancing from one step to another.

Risk Management

17. Using pictures or illustrations, explain the objectives and procedures of prophylactic taping, padding, and bandaging, as appropriate, for the injuries in list G.

18. Demonstrate or explain procedures for preventing each injury in list G.

References

AAOS 1999 (pp. 144-167, 198-218)

Anderson, Hall, and Martin 2000 (pp. 178-208)

Arnheim and Prentice 2000 (pp. 784-807)

Houglum 2001 (pp. 701-755)

Magee 1997 (pp. 101-147)

Shultz, Houglum, and Perrin 2000 (pp. 51-83)

Starkey and Ryan 2002 (pp. 369-394, 610-651)

Mastery and Demonstration

Practice and reinforce these competencies by reviewing your class notes and texts, observing peer teachers and certified/licensed professionals perform the skills, discussing the competencies with peer teachers and certified/licensed professionals, practicing alone and with a peer, and then demonstrating proficiency to a peer teacher. Finally, demonstrate your proficiency to an ACI.

Approved by (date and signature)

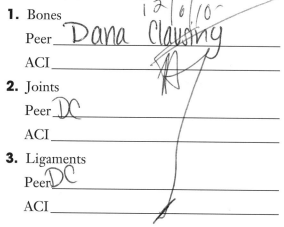

1. Bones

Peer _Dana Clausing_

ACI _____

2. Joints

Peer _DC_

ACI _____

3. Ligaments

Peer _DC_

ACI _____

4. Muscles

Peer _DC_____

ACI _____

5. Other structures

Peer _DC_____

ACI _____

6. History

Peer _DC_____

ACI _____

7. Special Tests

- Valsalva's maneuver

  Peer _DC_____

  ACI _____

- Distraction/compression

  Peer _DC_____

  ACI _____

- Spurling's test

  Peer _DC_____

  ACI _____

- Shoulder depression

  Peer _DC_____

  ACI _____

- Vertebral artery test

  Peer _DC_____

  ACI _____

- Brachial tension test

  Peer _DC_____

  ACI _____

- Tinel's sign

  Peer _DC_____

  ACI _____

- Upper extremity neurological evaluation

  Peer _DC_____

  ACI _____

8-18. Complete competencies 8-18 for the injuries or conditions in list G:

- Cervical dislocation

  Peer _____

  ACI _____

- Cervical subluxation

  Peer _____

  ACI _____

- Cervical sprain

  Peer _____

  ACI _____

- Cervical strain

  Peer _____

  ACI _____

- Neck contusion

  Peer _____

  ACI _____

- Neck burner

  Peer _____

  ACI _____

- Neck muscle atrophy

  Peer _____

  ACI _____

- Vertebral fracture

  Peer _____

  ACI _____

- Head and neck posture

  Peer _____

  ACI _____

- Intervertebral disc herniation

  Peer _____

  ACI _____

- Nerve root compression

  Peer _____

  ACI _____

- Spinal cord ischemia

  Peer_____

  ACI_____

- Torticollis

  Peer_____

  ACI_____

- Brachial plexus neuropathy

  Peer_____

  ACI_____

- Neurovascular dysfunction

  Peer_____

  ACI_____

- Vertebral artery occlusion

  Peer_____

  ACI_____

Comments

Specific Injury Management

Head and Facial Injury Management

Objective

Develop and demonstrate the skills necessary to properly evaluate, care for, rehabilitate, and prevent head and facial injuries.

Anatomy and Conditions for This Module

A. Bones and Prominent Bony Features

- Skull
  - Parietal
  - Occipital
  - Frontal
  - Temporal
- Mastoid process
- Mandible
- Maxilla
- Nasal (both)
- Zygomatic arch
- Ethmoid
- Sphenid
- Teeth

B. Articulations

- Temporomandibular

C. Other Structures

- Nasal passages
- Auris
  - Aurice (pinna)
  - External auditory canal
  - Tympanic membrane
  - Ossicles
  - Cochlea
  - Semicircular canals
- Eye
  - Cornea
  - Lens
  - Iris
  - Anterior chamber
  - Posterior chamber
  - Conjuctiva
  - Retina

D. Special Tests

- Amnesia (retrograde or posttraumatic)
- Levels of consciousness
- Orientation (person, time, place orientation)
- Intracranial hematoma
- Balance and coordination
- Pupil and eye movements
- Pulse
- Blood pressure
- Facial postures
- Cranial nerves (e.g., eye motion, facial muscles)
- Cognitive tests (e.g., recall, serial 7s, digit span)
- Cerebellar function (e.g., Romberg's test, finger-to-nose test, heel-toe walking, heel-to-knee standing)
- Spinal nerve roots (e.g., upper quarter screen)

E. Injuries and Conditions

Head and Face
- Skull fracture
- Jaw fracture
- Scalp hematoma
- Facial laceration
- Concussion
- Intracranial bleeding
- Headache

Eye
- Foreign body in the eye
- Contact lens lost in the eye
- Lens or iris injury

- Orbital blowout fracture
- Conjunctivitis (pink eye)
- Corneal abrasion
- Corneal laceration
- Detached retina
- Hyphema (eye chamber hemorrhage)
- Stye

Ear

- Impacted cerumen
- Otitis externa (swimmer's ear)
- Otitis media
- Hematoma auris ("cauliflower ear")
- Ruptured eardrum
- Foreign body in the ear

Nose

- Deviated septum
- Epistaxis (nose bleed)
- Nasal fracture

Jaw, Mouth, and Tooth

- Gingivitis
- Mandibular fracture
- Maxilla fracture
- Periodontitis
- Temporomandibular joint (TMJ) dislocation
- TMJ dysfunction
- Tooth abscess
- Tooth extrusion
- Tooth fracture
- Tooth intrusion
- Tooth luxation

Competencies

Note: All procedures must be performed.

Anatomical Review and Assessment of Structural Integrity

1. Name and palpate each bone and bony structure in list A. Also, tell what differences you would expect to feel if the bone was fractured.

2. Palpate the TMJ. Then perform active and passive joint ROM tests using both qualitative and quantitative techniques (e.g., tape measure, goniometer, and inclinometer). Record

results of these tests using accepted forms and procedures.

3. Identify, and palpate as possible, each structure in list C.

Injury Assessment

4. Obtain the medical history of an athlete with a suspected head injury.

5. Demonstrate proper administration and interpretation of the special tests in list D.

6. Demonstrate how you would observe and identify the clinical signs and symptoms associated with the injuries and conditions in list E.

7. Explain and demonstrate the mechanisms by which each injury in list E occurs. Name the three sports in which each injury is most likely to occur and explain any differences among the injury occurrences and mechanisms in those sports.

8. Demonstrate appropriate sensory, circulatory, and neurological tests for the injuries in list E.

9. Palpate and assess the integrity of the bones and soft tissues associated with each injury in list E.

10. Demonstrate functional and activity-specific tests to determine the integrity of each structure involved in each injury in list E.

Injury Management

11. Explain and demonstrate the appropriate immediate care procedures for each injury in list E. Explain the objectives and criteria for progressing for each step in the procedure.

12. Demonstrate a complete rehabilitation program for each injury in list E. As you proceed, explain the objectives and procedures of each step in the program. Explain the measurement criteria for advancing from one step to another.

Risk Management

13. Using pictures or illustrations, explain the objectives and procedures of prophylactic taping, padding, and bandaging, as appropriate, for the injuries in list E.

14. Demonstrate or explain procedures for preventing each injury in list E.

References

AAOS 1999 (pp. 170-195)

Anderson, Hall, and Martin 2000 (pp. 178-208)

Arnheim and Prentice 2000 (pp. 797-815)

Magee 1997 (pp. 53-98)

Shultz, Houglum, and Perrin 2000 (pp. 345-399, 453-458)

Starkey and Ryan 2002 (pp. 567-608)

Mastery and Demonstration

Practice and reinforce these competencies by reviewing your class notes and texts, observing peer teachers and certified/licensed professionals perform the skills, discussing the competencies with peer teachers and certified/licensed professionals, practicing alone and with a peer, and then demonstrating proficiency to a peer teacher. Finally, demonstrate your proficiency to an ACI.

Approved by (date and signature)

1. Bones

Peer_____

ACI_____

2. Joints

Peer_____

ACI_____

3. Other structures

Peer_____

ACI_____

4. History

Peer_____

ACI_____

5. Special Tests

- Amnesia

    Peer_____

    ACI_____

- Levels of consciousness

    Peer_____

    ACI_____

- Orientation

    Peer_____

    ACI_____

- Intracranial hematoma

    Peer_____

    ACI_____

- Balance and coordination

    Peer_____

    ACI_____

- Pupil and eye movements

    Peer_____

    ACI_____

- Pulse

    Peer_____

    ACI_____

- Blood pressure

    Peer_____

    ACI_____

- Facial postures

    Peer_____

    ACI_____

- Cranial nerves

    Peer_____

    ACI_____

- Cognitive tests

    Peer_____

    ACI_____

- Cerebellar function

    Peer_____

    ACI_____

- Spinal nerve roots

    Peer_____

    ACI_____

6-14. Complete competencies 6-14 for the injuries or conditions in list E:

Head and Face

- Skull fracture

  Peer_____

  ACI_____

- Jaw fracture

  Peer_____

  ACI_____

- Scalp hematoma

  Peer_____

  ACI_____

- Facial laceration

  Peer_____

  ACI_____

- Concussion

  Peer_____

  ACI_____

- Intracranial bleeding

  Peer_____

  ACI_____

- Headache

  Peer_____

  ACI_____

Eye

- Foreign body in eye

  Peer_____

  ACI_____

- Contact lens lost in eye

  Peer_____

  ACI_____

- Lens or iris injury

  Peer_____

  ACI_____

- Orbital blowout fracture

  Peer_____

  ACI_____

- Conjunctivitis

  Peer_____

  ACI_____

- Corneal abrasion

  Peer_____

  ACI_____

- Corneal laceration

  Peer_____

  ACI_____

- Detached retina

  Peer_____

  ACI_____

- Hyphema

  Peer_____

  ACI_____

- Stye

  Peer_____

  ACI_____

Ear

- Impacted cerumen

  Peer_____

  ACI_____

- Otitis externa

  Peer_____

  ACI_____

- Otitis media

  Peer_____

  ACI_____

- Hematoma auris

  Peer_____

  ACI_____

- Ruptured eardrum

  Peer_____

  ACI_____

- Foreign body in the ear

  Peer_____

  ACI_____

Nose
- Deviated septum

    Peer_____

    ACI_____

- Epistaxis

    Peer_____

    ACI_____

- Nasal fracture

    Peer_____

    ACI_____

Jaw, Mouth, and Tooth
- Gingivitis

    Peer_____

    ACI_____

- Mandibular fracture

    Peer_____

    ACI_____

- Maxilla fracture

    Peer_____

    ACI_____

- Periodontitis

    Peer_____

    ACI_____

- TMJ dislocation

    Peer_____

    ACI_____

- TMJ dysfunction

    Peer_____

    ACI_____

- Tooth abscess

    Peer_____

    ACI_____

- Tooth extrusion

    Peer_____

    ACI_____

- Tooth fracture

    Peer_____

    ACI_____

- Tooth intrusion

    Peer_____

    ACI_____

- Tooth luxation

    Peer_____

    ACI_____

Comments

Management of Simple Dermatological Conditions

Objective

Develop and demonstrate the skills necessary to properly evaluate, care for, and prevent simple dermatological conditions.

Conditions for This Module

- Abscess
- Acne vulgaris
- Blister
- Carbuncle
- Cellulitis
- Molluscum contagiosum
- Dermatitis
- Eczema
- Folliculitis
- Frostbite
- Furunculosis
- Herpes simplex
- Tinea versicolor
- Pediculosis
- Herpes zoster
- Hives
- Impetigo
- Psoriasis
- Ringworm
- Scabies
- Sebaceous cyst
- Tinea cruris
- Tinea pedis
- Urticaria
- Verruca plantaris
- Verruca vulgaris
- Tinea capitis

Competencies

1. Describe, with the use of pictures, the structure of the skin (including all the layers).

2. Describe, with the use of pictures if necessary, the signs, symptoms, and predisposing conditions associated with the diseases and conditions listed in this module. If any is more prevalent in specific sports, identify those sports.

3. Explain the impact each condition listed has on sports participation.

4. Explain and demonstrate the appropriate management procedures for each condition.

5. Demonstrate or explain procedures for preventing each condition.

References

AAOS 1999 (pp. 560-578)

Anderson, Hall, and Martin 2000 (pp. 637-655)

Arnheim and Prentice 2000 (pp. 817-843)

Magee 1997 (pp. 152-172)

Pfeiffer and Mangus 1998 (pp. 227-239)

Shultz, Houglum, and Perrin 2000 (pp. 408-419)

Starkey and Ryan 2002 (pp. 704-717)

Mastery and Demonstration

Practice and reinforce these competencies by reviewing your class notes and texts, observing peer teachers and certified/licensed professionals perform the skills, discussing the competencies with peer teachers and certified/licensed professionals, practicing alone and with a peer, and then demonstrating proficiency to a peer teacher. Finally, demonstrate your proficiency to an ACI.

Module J14—Management of Simple Dermatological Conditions (continued)

1. Skin structure

Peer _____

ACI _____

2-5. Complete competencies 2-5 for the following conditions:

- Abscess

    Peer _____

    ACI _____

- Acne vulgaris

    Peer _____

    ACI _____

- Blister

    Peer _____

    ACI _____

- Carbuncle

    Peer _____

    ACI _____

- Cellulitis

    Peer _____

    ACI _____

- Molluscum

    Peer _____

    ACI _____

- Dermatitis

    Peer _____

    ACI _____

- Eczema

    Peer _____

    ACI _____

- Folliculitis

    Peer _____

    ACI _____

- Frostbite

    Peer _____

    ACI _____

- Furunculosis

    Peer _____

    ACI _____

- Herpes simplex

    Peer _____

    ACI _____

- Tinea versicolor

    Peer _____

    ACI _____

- Pediculosis

    Peer _____

    ACI _____

- Herpes zoster

    Peer _____

    ACI _____

- Hives

    Peer _____

    ACI _____

- Impetigo

    Peer _____

    ACI _____

- Psoriasis

    Peer _____

    ACI _____

- Ringworm

    Peer _____

    ACI _____

- Scabies

    Peer _____

    ACI _____

- Sebaceous cysts

    Peer _____

    ACI _____

- Tinea cruris

    Peer _____

    ACI _____

- Tinea pedis

  Peer_____

  ACI_____

- Urticaria

  Peer_____

  ACI_____

- Verruca plantaris

  Peer_____

  ACI_____

- Verruca vulgaris

  Peer_____

  ACI_____

- Tinea capitis

  Peer_____

  ACI_____

Comments

Management of Common Syndromes and Diseases

Objective

Develop and demonstrate the skills necessary to properly evaluate, care for, and prevent common syndromes and diseases.

Syndromes and Diseases for This Module Description s/s

- Diabetes I + II
- Hyperthyroidism
- Hypothyroidism
- Pancreatitis
- Infectious mononucleosis
- Measles
- Mumps
- Epilepsy
- Syncope —
- Reflex sympathetic dystrophy —
- Meningitis
- Iron-deficiency anemia (systemic)
- Sickle cell anemia (systemic)
- Lyme disease —
- Apend

Competencies

1. Describe, with the use of pictures if necessary, the signs, symptoms, and predisposing conditions associated with the following syndromes and diseases. Tell how each condition affects athletes' performances in football, basketball, baseball/softball, track and field, and two other sports.

2. Explain, and demonstrate if possible, the appropriate management procedures for each condition listed in this module. Explain the objectives and criteria for progressing for each step in the procedure.

3. Explain guidelines for participation (practice and games) for athletes with each condition.

4. Demonstrate or explain procedures for preventing each condition.

References

AAOS 1999 (pp. 672-682)

Anderson, Hall, and Martin 2000 (pp. 550-572, 584-602)

Arnheim and Prentice 2000 (pp. 844-868)

Shultz, Houglum, and Perrin 2000 (pp. 430-434, 449-453)

Starkey and Ryan 2002 (pp. 684-697)

Mastery and Demonstration

Practice and reinforce these competencies by reviewing your class notes and texts, observing peer teachers and certified/licensed professionals perform the skills, discussing the competencies with peer teachers and certified/licensed professionals, practicing alone and with a peer, and then demonstrating proficiency to a peer teacher. Finally, demonstrate your proficiency to an ACI.

Approved by (date and signature)

1-4. Complete competencies 1-4 for the following symptoms or diseases:

- Diabetes
  Peer_____
  ACI_____

- Hyperthyroidism
  Peer_____
  ACI_____

- Hypothyroidism
  Peer_____
  ACI_____

- Pancreatitis

  Peer_____

  ACI_____

- Infectious mononucleosis

  Peer_____

  ACI_____

- Measles

  Peer_____

  ACI_____

- Mumps

  Peer_____

  ACI_____

- Epilepsy

  Peer_____

  ACI_____

- Syncope

  Peer_____

  ACI_____

- Reflex sympathetic dystrophy

  Peer_____

  ACI_____

- Meningitis

  Peer_____

  ACI_____

- Iron-deficiency anemia

  Peer_____

  ACI_____

- Sickle cell anemia

  Peer_____

  ACI_____

- Lyme disease

  Peer_____

  ACI_____

Comments

Specific Injury Management

Management of Common Viral and Respiratory Tract Conditions and Disorders

Objective

Develop and demonstrate the skills necessary to properly evaluate, care for, and prevent common viral and respiratory tract conditions and disorders.

Conditions and Disorders for This Module

Do All
S/S
Tx

- Common cold
- Influenza
- Laryngitis
- Pharyngitis
- Rhinitis
- Sinusitis
- Tetanus
- Tonsillitis
- Asthma
- Bronchitis
- Hyperventilation
- Hay fever
- Pneumonia
- Upper respiratory infection (URI)

Competencies

1. Describe, with the use of pictures if necessary, the signs, symptoms, and predisposing conditions associated with the conditions and disorders listed in this module. Tell how each condition affects athletes' performances in football, basketball, baseball/softball, track and field, and two other sports.

2. Explain, and demonstrate if possible, the appropriate management procedures for each condition. Explain the objectives and criteria for progressing for each step in the procedure.

3. Explain guidelines for participation (practice and games) for athletes with each condition.

4. Demonstrate or explain procedures for preventing each condition listed.

References

AAOS 1999 (pp. 654-664, 714-735)

Anderson, Hall, and Martin 2000 (pp. 550-557)

Arnheim and Prentice 2000 (pp. 832, 847-855)

Shultz, Houglum, and Perrin 2000 (pp. 419-430)

Starkey and Ryan 2002 (pp. 680-683)

A comprehensive medical dictionary

Mastery and Demonstration

Practice and reinforce these competencies by reviewing your class notes and texts, observing peer teachers and certified/licensed professionals perform the skills, discussing the competencies with peer teachers and certified/licensed professionals, practicing alone and with a peer, and then demonstrating proficiency to a peer teacher. Finally, demonstrate your proficiency to an ACI.

Approved by (date and signature)

1-4. Complete competencies 1-4 for the following conditions and disorders.

- Common cold

  Peer_____

  ACI_____

- Influenza

  Peer_____

  ACI_____

- Laryngitis

  Peer_____

  ACI_____

- Pharyngitis

  Peer_____

  ACI_____

- Rhinitis

  Peer_____

  ACI_____

- Sinusitis

  Peer_____

  ACI_____

- Tetanus

  Peer_____

  ACI_____

- Tonsillitis

  Peer_____

  ACI_____

- Asthma

  Peer_____

  ACI_____

- Bronchitis

  Peer_____

  ACI_____

- Hyperventilation

  Peer_____

  ACI_____

- Hay fever

  Peer_____

  ACI_____

- Pneumonia

  Peer_____

  ACI_____

- URI

  Peer_____

  ACI_____

Comments

Management of Common Cardiovascular and Gastrointestinal Tract Conditions and Disorders

Objective

Develop and demonstrate the skills necessary to properly evaluate, care for, and prevent common cardiovascular and gastrointestinal tract conditions and disorders.

Conditions and Disorders ~Do All~ for This Module

- Hypertension
- Hypotension
- Hypertrophic myocardiopathy
- Migraine headache
- Sudden death
- Appendicitis
- Colitis
- Constipation
- Diarrhea
- Esophageal reflux
- Gastritis
- Gastroenteritis
- Indigestion
- Ulcer
- Irritable bowel syndrome

Competencies

1. Describe, with the use of pictures if necessary, the signs, symptoms, and predisposing conditions associated with the conditions and disorders listed in this module. Tell how each condition affects athletes' performances in football, basketball, baseball/softball, track and field, and two other sports.

2. Explain, and demonstrate if possible, the appropriate management procedures for each condition. Explain the objectives and criteria for progressing for each step in the procedure.

3. Explain guidelines for participation (practice and games) for athletes with each condition.

4. Demonstrate or explain procedures for preventing each condition.

References

Anderson, Hall, and Martin 2000 (pp. 589-593)

Arnheim and Prentice 2000 (pp. 771-797, 857-858)

Shultz, Houglum, and Perrin 2000 (pp. 421-442)

Starkey and Ryan 2002 (pp. 667-679, 704-705)

A comprehensive medical dictionary

Mastery and Demonstration

Practice and reinforce these competencies by reviewing your class notes and texts, observing peer teachers and certified/licensed professionals perform the skills, discussing the competencies with peer teachers and certified/licensed professionals, practicing alone and with a peer, and then demonstrating proficiency to a peer teacher. Finally, demonstrate your proficiency to an ACI.

Approved by (date and signature)

1-4. Complete competencies 1-4 for the following conditions and disorders:

- Hypertension
  Peer_____
  ACI_____

- Hypotension
  Peer_____
  ACI_____

- Hypertrophic myocardiopathy

  Peer_____

  ACI_____

- Migraine

  Peer_____

  ACI_____

- Sudden death

  Peer_____

  ACI_____

- Appendicitis

  Peer_____

  ACI_____

- Colitis

  Peer_____

  ACI_____

- Constipation

  Peer_____

  ACI_____

- Diarrhea

  Peer_____

  ACI_____

- Esophageal reflux

  Peer_____

  ACI_____

- Gastritis

  Peer_____

  ACI_____

- Gastroenteritis

  Peer_____

  ACI_____

- Indigestion

  Peer_____

  ACI_____

- Ulcer

  Peer_____

  ACI_____

- Irritable bowel

  Peer_____

  ACI_____

Comments

Management of Common Genitourinary, Gynecological, and Sexually Related Conditions, Disorders, and Diseases

Objective

Develop and demonstrate the skills necessary to properly evaluate, care for, and prevent common genitourinary, gynecological, and sexually-related conditions, disorders, and diseases.

Conditions and Disorders for This Module

- Kidney stones
- Spermatic cord torsion
- Candidiasis
- Urethritis
- Urinary tract infection
✗ Hydrocele
- Hemorrhoid
- Varicocele
- Amenorrhea
- Dysmenorrhea
✗ Oligomenorrhea
- Pelvic inflammatory disease
- Vaginitis
- HIV/acquired immunodeficiency syndrome (AIDS)
- Hepatitis
- Chlamydia
- Genital warts
- Gonorrhea
- Syphilis

Competencies

1. Describe, with the use of pictures if necessary, the signs, symptoms, and predisposing conditions associated with the conditions, diseases, and disorders listed in this module. Tell how each condition affects athletes' performances in football, basketball, baseball/softball, track and field, and two other sports.

2. Explain, and demonstrate if possible, the appropriate management procedures for each condition listed. Explain the objectives and criteria for progressing for each step in the procedure.

3. Explain guidelines for participation (practice and games) for athletes with each condition.

4. Demonstrate or explain procedures for preventing each condition.

References

Anderson, Hall, and Martin 2000 (pp. 578-583, 604-609)

Arnheim and Prentice 2000 (pp. 256-272)

Shultz, Houglum, and Perrin 2000 (pp. 442-446)

Starkey and Ryan 2002 (pp. 686-691)

Mastery and Demonstration

Practice and reinforce these competencies by reviewing your class notes and texts, observing peer teachers and certified/licensed professionals perform the skills, discussing the competencies with peer teachers and certified/licensed professionals, practicing alone and with a peer, and then demonstrating proficiency to a peer teacher. Finally, demonstrate your proficiency to an ACI.

Approved by (date and signature)

1-4. Complete competencies 1-4 for the following conditions, disorders, and diseases:

- Kidney stones

  Peer _____

  ACI _____

Module J18—Management of Common Genitourinary, Gynecological, and Sexually Related Conditions, Disorders, and Diseases (continued)

- Spermatic cord torsion

  Peer _____

  ACI _____

- Candidiasis

  Peer _____

  ACI _____

- Urethritis

  Peer _____

  ACI _____

- Urinary tract infection

  Peer _____

  ACI _____

- Hydrocele

  Peer _____

  ACI _____

- Hemorrhoid

  Peer _____

  ACI _____

- Varicocele

  Peer _____

  ACI _____

- Amenorrhea

  Peer _____

  ACI _____

- Dysmenorrhea

  Peer _____

  ACI _____

- Oligomenorrhea

  Peer _____

  ACI _____

- Pelvic inflammatory disease

  Peer _____

  ACI _____

- Vaginitis

  Peer _____

  ACI _____

- HIV/AIDS

  Peer _____

  ACI _____

- Hepatitis

  Peer _____

  ACI _____

- Chlamydia

  Peer _____

  ACI _____

- Genital warts

  Peer _____

  ACI _____

- Gonorrhea

  Peer _____

  ACI _____

- Syphilis

  Peer _____

  ACI _____

Comments

O/P Examination 2

Objectives

Demonstrate your mastery of Levels 1, 2, and 3 skills and continue your preparation for the NATA O/P examination.

Competencies

Complete your program's comprehensive O/P examination with a score of at least 85%.

References

Individual module references

Mastery and Demonstration

Date taken _____

Score _____

Approved by _____

Reexamination _____

Score _____

Approved by _____

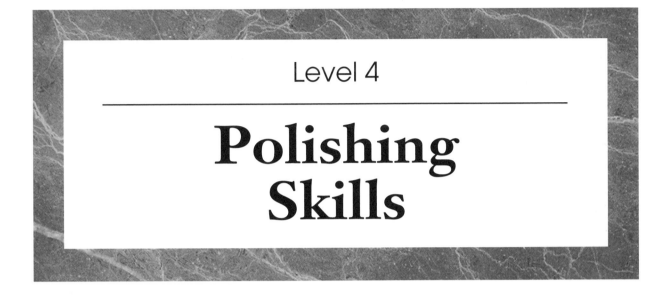

Level 4

Polishing Skills

By now students should have demonstrated the ability to perform all of the psychomotor skills necessary for an entry-level athletic trainer. Are they proficient? More so in some skills than others. Are they ready to tackle the world? Not yet, but they should be close. Level 4 modules are designed to help athletic training students polish their psychomotor skills and develop and demonstrate proficiency in communication, administration, and presentation skills.

Team Athletic Training Student

Objective

Polish your skills as you serve as the "head" athletic training student for a specific athletic team during its entire sport season.

Competencies

Work with a specific athletic team during its entire sport season (preseason conditioning through off-season conditioning). Among other things, do the following:

1. Assist with the physical examination of athletes.

2. Assist with evaluating the team's level of conditioning.

3. Inspect the athletic training clinic for compliance with safety and sanitary standards.

4. Be a team leader in a mock removal from the field or court of an athlete with a possible cervical injury.

5. Inventory equipment and supplies.

6. Prepare an equipment and supply purchase request for the next season, based on your inventory.

7. Supervise rotating Level 1 and Level 3 students assigned to your team as directed by the head staff athletic trainer for your team.

Mastery and Demonstration

Obtain the signature of an ACI (and the date) when you have completed this module.

ACI _____

Comments

Clinical Capstone Experience

Objective

Expand your horizons and continue to polish your skills.

Competencies

Serve as an athletic training student with another institution (high school, another college, professional team, or a sports medicine clinic) for at least 6 weeks or for an athletic team at your university during their entire sport season, including preseason conditioning, regular season, and off-season conditioning. (Note: This must be in addition to and following Module X12.)

Mastery and Demonstration

Obtain the signature of an ACI (and the date) when you have completed this module.

ACI _____

Comments

Supervise/Teach Level 3 Students

Objective

Teach Level 3 skills, assess mastery of those skills by Level 3 students, and deepen your own understanding and mastery of those skills.

Competencies

1. Peer teach at least four different Level 3 students and at least 20 Level 3 modules. This includes reviewing material with the students, offering suggestions and corrections as necessary as they practice the skills, and then assessing their mastery of the skill when appropriate. Students must practice the skills long enough that they become proficient with them before assessment. Refer often to references and teaching aids.

2. Discuss your peer teaching experience with a faculty athletic trainer or clinical instructor.

References

Your athletic training department library and the references to individual Level 3 modules

Mastery and Demonstration

1. Peer teaching

Name of Student	Module	Review Date	Approval Date
1. _____	_____	_____	_____
2. _____	_____	_____	_____
3. _____	_____	_____	_____
4. _____	_____	_____	_____
5. _____	_____	_____	_____
6. _____	_____	_____	_____
7. _____	_____	_____	_____
8. _____	_____	_____	_____
9. _____	_____	_____	_____
10. _____	_____	_____	_____
11. _____	_____	_____	_____
12. _____	_____	_____	_____
13. _____	_____	_____	_____
14. _____	_____	_____	_____
15. _____	_____	_____	_____
16. _____	_____	_____	_____
17. _____	_____	_____	_____
18. _____	_____	_____	_____

Name of Student	Module	Review Date	Approval Date
19. _____	_____	_____	_____
20. _____	_____	_____	_____
21. _____	_____	_____	_____
22. _____	_____	_____	_____
23. _____	_____	_____	_____
24. _____	_____	_____	_____
25. _____	_____	_____	_____
26. _____	_____	_____	_____
27. _____	_____	_____	_____
28. _____	_____	_____	_____
29. _____	_____	_____	_____
30. _____	_____	_____	_____

2. Task completed and discussed (date)

_____

Approved by

_____

Comments

Administer Comprehensive O/P Examination

Objective

Teach Level 3 skills, assess their mastery of those skills by Level 3 students, and deepen your own understanding and mastery of those skills.

Competency

Assist your program director examine Level 3 students by serving as an examiner for at least five different O/P examinations.

Mastery and Demonstration

Serve as examiner.

Person examined	Date
1.	
2.	
3.	
4.	
5.	
6.	
7.	
8.	
9.	
10.	

Approved by

ACI

Comments

Write O/P Questions

Objective

Refine your teaching skills.

Competency

In consultation with your athletic training program director, select a subject and then write an O/P examination question. Follow the format of questions used by your athletic training program.

References

Use references specific to the content of the question

Mastery and Demonstration

Give a copy of the question to your athletic training program director.

Approved by

ACI_____

Comments

Update Reference Material

Objective

Help update your athletic training clinic reference library, and deepen your own understanding and mastery of those skills.

Competency

Search current literature (texts or professional journals) for two new module references. These may be for the same module or for two different modules. Both references must offer specific information to help students master the skills (competencies) of the module.

References

Your university or hospital libraries

Mastery and Demonstration

Give a copy of the complete reference, with full bibliographic citation, to your athletic training program director.

Approved by

ACI _____

Comments

Healthcare Communication

Objective

Demonstrate your ability to communicate appropriately with a diversity of individuals.

Competencies

Demonstrate appropriate communication skills to achieve the following:

1. Calm, reassure, and explain a potentially catastrophic injury to an injured adult or child, athletic personnel, or family member.

2. Effectively communicate and work with physicians, emergency medical technicians, and other members of the allied healthcare community and sports medicine team.

3. Appropriately communicate with athletic personnel and family members.

4. Use ethnic and cultural sensitivity in all aspects of communication.

5. Communicate with diverse community populations.

References

AAOS 1999 (pp. 5-16)

Pfeiffer and Mangus 1998 (pp. 21-28)

Rankin and Ingersoll 2001 (pp. 20-35)

Ray 2000 (pp. 10-21)

Starkey and Ryan 2002 (pp. 26-28)

Mastery and Demonstration

Practice and reinforce these competencies by reviewing your class notes and texts, observing peer teachers and certified/licensed professionals perform the skills, discussing the competencies with peer teachers and certified/licensed professionals, practicing alone and with a peer, and then demonstrating proficiency to a peer teacher. Finally, demonstrate your proficiency to an ACI.

Approved by (date and signature)

1. Calm/reassure

   Peer _____

   ACI _____

2. Other healthcare workers

   Peer _____

   ACI _____

3. Athletic personnel

   Peer _____

   ACI _____

4. Ethnic sensitivity

   Peer _____

   ACI _____

5. Diverse community

   Peer _____

   ACI _____

Comments

Substance Abuse

Objective

Demonstrate your ability to assist a substance-abusing athlete find professional help.

Competencies

1. Simulate intervention with an individual who has a substance abuse problem, such as alcohol, tobacco, stimulants, nutritional supplements, steroids, marijuana, and narcotics, and recommend appropriate referral.

2. Simulate a confidential conversation with a healthcare professional concerning suspected substance abuse by an athlete.

3. Prepare a list of available community-based resources to which you can refer athletes for substance abuse counseling.

References

AAOS 1999 (pp. 770-795)

Arnheim and Prentice 2000 (pp. 432-441)

Mastery and Demonstration

Practice and reinforce these competencies by reviewing your class notes and texts, observing peer teachers and certified/licensed professionals perform the skills, discussing the competencies with peer teachers and certified/licensed professionals, practicing alone and with a peer, and then demonstrating proficiency to a peer teacher. Finally, demonstrate your proficiency to an ACI.

Approved by (date and signature)

1. Individual

Peer_____

ACI_____

2. Professional

Peer_____

ACI_____

3. Resources

Peer_____

ACI_____

Comments

Psychosocial Intervention

Objective

Locate the available community-based resources to which you can refer athletes for psychosocial intervention.

Competencies

1. Prepare a list of community-based resources for psychosocial intervention for your athletes. In this list, include the professionals' names, specialties, addresses, and phone numbers.

References

Phone book

Arnheim and Prentice 2000 (pp. 256-272)

Mastery and Demonstration

Practice and reinforce these competencies by reviewing your class notes and texts, observing peer teachers and certified/licensed professionals perform the skills, discussing the competencies with peer teachers and certified/licensed professionals, practicing alone and with a peer, and then demonstrating proficiency to a peer teacher. Finally, demonstrate your proficiency to an ACI.

Approved by (date and signature)

1. List

Peer_____

ACI_____

Comments

Information and Data Management Tools

Objective

Demonstrate your ability to access information and manage data using contemporary multimedia, computer equipment, and software.

Competencies

Demonstrate your ability to use the following types of computer software:

1. Word processing software

2. File management systems

3. Spreadsheets

4. World Wide Web

5. Communication (e-mail)

6. Budgeting software

7. Injury tracking software

References

Faculty of your institution

Credit or noncredit classes

Rankin and Ingersoll 2001 (pp. 298-303)

Ray 2000 (pp. 179-188)

Mastery and Demonstration

Practice and reinforce these competencies by reviewing your class notes and texts, observing peer teachers and certified/licensed professionals perform the skills, discussing the competencies with peer teachers and certified/licensed professionals, practicing alone and with a peer, and then demonstrating proficiency to a peer teacher. Finally, demonstrate your proficiency to an ACI.

Approved by (date and signature)

1. Word processing

   Peer _____

   ACI _____

2. File management

   Peer _____

   ACI _____

3. Spreadsheet

   Peer _____

   ACI _____

4. World Wide Web

   Peer _____

   ACI _____

5. E-mail

   Peer _____

   ACI _____

6. Budgeting

   Peer _____

   ACI _____

7. Injury tracking

   Peer _____

   ACI _____

Comments

Preparticipation Medical/Physical Examination

Objective

Understand the organization and administration of a preparticipation medical/physical examination.

Competencies

1. Discuss the following aspects of an upcoming preparticipation medical/physical examination at your institution:

   a. Governing principles/rational

   b. Goals

   c. Legal ramifications

   d. Forms used to evaluate athletes' medical history

   e. Appropriate medical and musculoskeletal examination tests

   f. Professionals involved in exam

2. Assist in organizing and administering a preparticipation medical/physical examination at your institution by performing tasks assigned by your clinical instructor.

References

Pfeiffer and Mangus 1998 (pp. 41-44, 313-314)

Rankin and Ingersoll 2001 (pp. 232-246)

Ray 2000 (pp. 255-283)

Magee 1997 (pp. 758-775)

Athletic training clinical staff

Mastery and Demonstration

Practice and reinforce these competencies by reviewing your class notes and texts, observing peer teachers and certified/licensed professionals perform the skills, discussing the competencies with peer teachers and certified/licensed professionals, practicing alone and with a peer, and then demonstrating proficiency to a peer teacher. Finally, demonstrate your proficiency to an ACI.

Approved by (date and signature)

1. Discuss preparticipation examination

   Peer _____

   ACI _____

2. Take part in preparticipation examination

   Peer _____

   ACI _____

Comments

Revise Policies and Procedures Manual

Objective

Develop your administrative skills.

Competency

In consultation with your head athletic trainer, select a section of your department's policies and procedures manual that needs updating. Revise the section and get it approved by your head athletic trainer.

References

Rankin and Ingersoll 2001 (pp. 88-403)

Ray 2000 (pp. 22-103)

Athletic training clinical staff

Mastery and Demonstration

Provide a copy of the completed update to your head athletic trainer.

Peer _____

ACI _____

Comments

Administrative Plans

Objective

Demonstrate the ability to develop administrative plans for an athletic training clinical department.

Competency

Demonstrate the ability to develop administrative plans that include but are not limited to the following:

1. Risk management

2. Developing policies and procedures

3. Developing a budget (expendable and capital)

4. Addressing facility hazards

References

Rankin and Ingersoll 2001 (pp. 88-103, 206-231)

Ray 2000 (pp. 22-128)

Mastery and Demonstration

Practice and reinforce these competencies by reviewing your class notes and texts, observing peer teachers and certified/licensed professionals perform the skills, discussing the competencies with peer teachers and certified/licensed professionals, practicing alone and with a peer, and then demonstrating proficiency to a peer teacher. Finally, demonstrate your proficiency to an ACI.

Approved by (date and signature)

1. Risk management

Peer_____

ACI_____

2. Policies and procedures

Peer_____

ACI_____

3. Budget

Peer_____

ACI_____

4. Facility hazards

Peer_____

ACI_____

Comments

Write down some changes in the facility what I would make + reasons why

Facility Design

Objective

Develop the ability to design athletic training facilities.

Competency

1. Design an athletic training facility that includes at least the following components:

  a. Basic floor plan design, detailed enough to show where furniture and equipment will be located

  b. Basic rehabilitation and treatment areas

  c. Facility evacuation plan

References

Rankin and Ingersoll 2001 (pp. 104-122)

Ray 2000 (pp. 130-156)

Mastery and Demonstration

Practice and reinforce these competencies by reviewing your class notes and texts, observing peer teachers and certified/licensed professionals perform the skills, discussing the competencies with peer teachers and certified/licensed professionals, practicing alone and with a peer, and then demonstrating proficiency to a peer teacher. Finally, demonstrate your proficiency to an ACI.

Approved by (date and signature)

1. Design

Peer_____

ACI_____

Comments

Interpret Current Literature

Objective

Demonstrate the ability to interpret basic professional literature.

Competencies

1. Demonstrate the ability to interpret a case study by reading about how case studies should be written. Next, read a specific case study published in the past 5 years in a professional journal. Then discuss the following:

  a. Describe the major sections of a properly written case study and the types of information that are in each section. Did the case study you read follow this procedure?

  b. Describe in general how a case study can help you provide better health care. What specific insights did this case provide you?

  c. Describe potential errors you could make when reading and interpreting a case study. How did you avoid these errors when reading this case study?

  d. What questions about the injury/illness presented in this case study did you think of while or after reading the case study? What strategies can you use to answer those questions?

2. Demonstrate the ability to interpret a literature review by reading about how literature reviews should be written. Next, read a specific literature review published in the past 5 years in a professional journal. Then discuss the following:

  a. Describe the major sections of a properly written literature review and the types of information that are in each section. Did the literature review you read follow this procedure?

  b. Describe in general how a literature review can help you provide better health care. What specific insights did this case provide you?

  c. Describe potential errors you could make when reading and interpreting a literature review. How did you avoid these errors when reading this literature review?

  d. What questions about the injury/illness presented in the literature review did you think of while or after reading the literature review? What strategies can you use to answer those questions?

3. Discuss outcome measurements as used in healthcare research.

4. Discuss the role of statistical procedures in interpreting outcome measurements.

References

Authors Guide, *Journal of Athletic Training*

Any statistics text

Ingersoll 2002

Mastery and Demonstration

Practice and reinforce these competencies by reviewing your class notes and texts, observing peer teachers and certified/licensed professionals perform the skills, discussing the competencies with peer teachers and certified/licensed professionals, practicing alone and with a peer, and then demonstrating proficiency to a peer teacher. Finally, demonstrate your proficiency to an ACI.

Approved by (date and signature)

1. Case study

  Peer _____

  ACI _____

2. Literature review

  Peer _____

  ACI _____

3. Outcome measurements   **Comments**

Peer_____

ACI _____

4. Statistical procedures

Peer_____

ACI _____

Professional Presentation

Objective

Demonstrate your ability to make a professional presentation to others concerning athletic training.

Competencies

1. Write an outline for a 10-minute presentation of an athletic training topic to one of the following groups of professional acquaintances. Include in the outline potential visual aids.

a. Peer athletic trainers

b. Physicians

c. Parents

d. Athletic personnel

e. General public

f. Athletes and others involved in physical activity

2. Develop your outline into a computer-based presentation (such as PowerPoint or Corel Presentations), and make the presentation.

References

University audiovisual department

University faculty

Ingersoll 2002

Mastery and Demonstration

Practice and reinforce these competencies by reviewing your class notes and texts, observing peer teachers and certified/licensed professionals perform the skills, discussing the competencies with peer teachers and certified/licensed professionals, practicing alone and with a peer, and then demonstrating proficiency to a peer teacher. Finally, demonstrate your proficiency to an ACI.

Approved by (date and signature)

1. Outline

Peer _____

ACI _____

2. Presentation

Peer _____

ACI _____

Comments

Presenting Yourself to the Job Market

Objective

Prepare to sell yourself to a potential employer or graduate school.

Competencies

1. Visit your college placement bureau and discuss its services with a counselor.

2. Prepare a resume that outlines your professional preparation and experiences.

3. Write a letter of intent to apply for a professional position or a graduate program.

References

Rankin and Ingersoll 2001 (pp. 54-69)

Your college placement bureau

Mastery and Demonstration

Practice and reinforce these competencies by reviewing your class notes and texts, discussing the competencies with peer teachers and certified/licensed professionals, practicing alone and with a peer, and then demonstrating proficiency to a peer teacher. Finally, demonstrate your proficiency to an ACI.

Approved by (date and signature)

1. Placement

Peer_____

ACI_____

2. Resume

Peer_____

ACI_____

3. Letter

Peer_____

ACI_____

Comments

Appendix A

Master Files

Level 1: Introduction to the Clinic

Name _____

School phone_____   School address_____

Permanent phone _____   Permanent address_____

MODULE	DATE COMPLETED	EVALUATOR COMMENTS
Directed Clinical Experience		
X1 Athletic Training Observation	_____	_____
Athletic Training Clinic Operations		
A1 Administrative Policies and Procedures	_____	_____
A2 Injury Record Keeping	_____	_____
A3 Athletic Training Supplies	_____	_____
A4 Athletic Training Clinic Equipment—Small	_____	_____
A5 Athletic Training Clinic Equipment—Major	_____	_____
Acute Care of Injuries and Illnesses		
B1 Implement Emergency Action Plan	_____	_____
B2 Cardiopulmonary Resuscitation	_____	_____
B3 Choking, Hemorrhaging, and Shock	_____	_____
B4 Emergency Transportation	_____	_____
B5 Medical Services	_____	_____

MODULE	DATE COMPLETED	EVALUATOR COMMENTS
B6 Rest, Ice, Compression, Elevation, Support	_____	_____
B7 Open Wounds	_____	_____
B8 Universal Precautions Against Bloodborne Pathogens, Hepatitis, and Tuberculosis	_____	_____
B9 Environmental Injury/Illness	_____	_____
B10 Anaphylaxis and Asthma Attacks	_____	_____
B11 Poison Control Center	_____	_____

ADDITIONAL MODULES	DATE COMPLETED	EVALUATOR COMMENTS
_____	_____	_____
_____	_____	_____
_____	_____	_____
_____	_____	_____
_____	_____	_____
_____	_____	_____

Level 2: Basic Skills

Name _____

School phone_____   School address_____

Permanent phone _____   Permanent address_____

MODULE	DATE COMPLETED	EVALUATOR COMMENTS
Directed Clinical Experience		
X2 Athletic Training Clinic Student Staff	_____	_____
X3 Athletic Training Clinic Student Staff	_____	_____
Peer Teaching/Supervision		
T1 Teach Level 1 Athletic Training Students	_____	_____

MODULE	DATE COMPLETED	EVALUATOR COMMENTS
Taping, Wrapping, Bracing, and Padding		
C1 Ankle Taping, Wrapping, and Bracing	_____	_____
C2 Knee Taping, Wrapping, and Bracing	_____	_____
C3 Thigh and Lower Leg Taping, Wrapping, and Padding	_____	_____
C4 Foot Care, Taping, Wrapping, and Padding	_____	_____
C5 Hip and Abdomen Taping, Wrapping, and Bracing	_____	_____
C6 Shoulder Taping, Wrapping, and Bracing	_____	_____
C7 Elbow-to-Wrist Taping, Wrapping, and Bracing	_____	_____
C8 Hand and Finger Taping and Wrapping	_____	_____
C9 Head and Neck Padding and Bracing	_____	_____
Risk Management		
D1 Anthropometric Measurements and Screening Procedures	_____	_____
D2 Protective Equipment Fitting	_____	_____
D3 Developing Flexibility	_____	_____
D4 Strength Training	_____	_____
Basic Assessment and Evaluation		
E1 General Medical Assessment	_____	_____
E2 Postural Assessment	_____	_____
E3 Neurological Assessment	_____	_____
E4 Palpation	_____	_____
E5 Assessing Range of Motion	_____	_____
E6 Physical Performance Measurements	_____	_____

MODULE	DATE COMPLETED	EVALUATOR COMMENTS
Basic Pharmacology and Nutrition		
F1 Medication Resources	_____	_____
F2 Medication Policies and Procedures	_____	_____
F3 Basic Performance Nutrition	_____	_____
F4 Eating Disorders	_____	_____
Therapeutic Modalities		
G1 Whirlpool	_____	_____
G2 Moist Hot Packs	_____	_____
G3 Paraffin Bath	_____	_____
G4 Cryotherapy	_____	_____
G5 Cryokinetics	_____	_____
G6 Cryostretch	_____	_____
G7 Intermittent Compression Devices	_____	_____
G8 Ultrasound	_____	_____
G9 Diathermy	_____	_____
G10 Electrical Stimulation	_____	_____
G11 Therapeutic Massage	_____	_____
G12 Traction	_____	_____
Therapeutic Exercise		
H1 Rehabilitation Overview	_____	_____
H2 Rehabilitation Adherence and Motivation Techniques	_____	_____
H3 Range of Motion and Flexibility Exercises	_____	_____
H4 Joint Mobilization	_____	_____
H5 Isometric Resistance Exercises	_____	_____
H6 Isotonic Strength-Training Devices	_____	_____
H7 Daily Adjustable Progressive Exercise	_____	_____

MODULE	DATE COMPLETED	EVALUATOR COMMENTS
H8 Isokinetic Dynamometers	_____	_____
H9 Muscular Endurance	_____	_____
H10 Aquatic Therapy	_____	_____
H11 Neuromuscular Control and Coordination Exercises	_____	_____
H12 Muscular Speed Exercises	_____	_____
H13 Agility Exercises	_____	_____
H14 Plyometrics	_____	_____
H15 Cardiorespiratory Endurance	_____	_____
H16 Activity-Specific Skills	_____	_____

Examination

	DATE COMPLETED	EVALUATOR COMMENTS
O/P Examination (Level 1 and 2 skills)	_____	_____

ADDITIONAL MODULES	DATE COMPLETED	EVALUATOR COMMENTS
_____	_____	_____
_____	_____	_____
_____	_____	_____
_____	_____	_____

Level 3: Integration of Skills

Name _____

School phone_____ School address_____

Permanent phone _____ Permanent address_____

MODULE	DATE COMPLETED	EVALUATOR COMMENTS

Directed Clinical Experience (Team Athletic Training Staff)

	DATE COMPLETED	EVALUATOR COMMENTS
X4 Football Team Experience	_____	_____
X5 Basketball Team Experience	_____	_____

MODULE	DATE COMPLETED	EVALUATOR COMMENTS
X6 Men's Team Sport Experience		
X7 Women's Team Sport Experience		
X8 Men's Individual Sport Experience		
X9 Women's Individual Sport Experience		
X10 High School Experience		
X11 Sports Medicine Clinic Experience		

Peer Teaching/Supervision

T2 Supervise/Teach Level 2 Students		
T3 Administer O/P Exam 1		

Observe Surgery

I1 Surgical Observation		

Specific Injury Management

J1 Foot Injury Management		
J2 Ankle Injury Management		
J3 Lower Leg Injury Management		
J4 Knee Injury Management		
J5 Thigh Injury Management		
J6 Hip and Pelvic Injury Management		
J7 Thorax and Lumbar Spine Injury Management		
J8 Thorax and Abdominal Injury Management		
J9 Shoulder Injury Management		
J10 Arm and Elbow Injury Management		
J11 Wrist and Hand Injury Management		
J12 Cervical Spine Injury Management		
J13 Head and Facial Injury Management		

MODULE	DATE COMPLETED	EVALUATOR COMMENTS
J14 Management of Simple Dermatological Conditions	_____	_____
J15 Management of Common Syndromes and Diseases	_____	_____
J16 Management of Common Viral and Respiratory Tract Conditions and Disorders	_____	_____
J17 Management of Common Cardiovascular and Gastrointestinal Tract Conditions and Disorders	_____	_____
J18 Management of Common Genitourinary, Gynecological, and Sexually Related Conditions, Disorders, and Diseases	_____	_____

Examination

O/P Examination (Level 1, 2, and 3 skills)	_____	_____

ADDITIONAL MODULES	DATE COMPLETED	EVALUATOR COMMENTS
_____	_____	_____
_____	_____	_____
_____	_____	_____
_____	_____	_____
_____	_____	_____

Level 4: Polishing Skills

Name _____

School phone_____ School address_____

Permanent phone _____ Permanent address_____

MODULE	DATE COMPLETED	EVALUATOR COMMENTS
Directed Clinical Experience (Team Student Staff)		
X12 Team Athletic Training Student	_____	_____
X13 Clinical Capstone Experience	_____	_____

MODULE	DATE COMPLETED	EVALUATOR COMMENTS

Peer Teaching

T4 Supervise/Teach Level 3 Students

T5 Administer Comprehensive O/P Exam

T6 Write O/P Questions

T7 Update Reference Material

Communication

K1 Healthcare Communication

K2 Substance Abuse

K3 Psychosocial Intervention

Administration

L1 Information and Data Management Tools

L2 Preparticipation Medical/Physical
    Examination

L3 Revise Policies and Procedures Manual

L4 Administrative Plans

L5 Facility Design

Athletic Training Presentation

M1 Interpret Current Literature

M2 Professional Presentation

M3 Presenting Yourself to the Job Market

ADDITIONAL MODULES	DATE COMPLETED	EVALUATOR COMMENTS

Appendix B

Information for Customizing Modules

Following are examples of customizing 4 modules. The lists of records, supplies, equipment, and services are used by various universities for completing the modules. Your clinical supervisor will probably use a different list; these are given merely for illustration.

MODULE A2—Injury Record Keeping (page 15)

1. Daily treatment log
2. Individual treatment sheets
3. Injury/insurance record
4. Physician referral
5. Rehabilitation center referral
6. Medical history
7. Medical history update
8. Physician reports
9. Computerized injury/treatment report

MODULE A3—Athletic Training Supplies (page 17)

- Triple antibiotic ointment, 1-ounce tube
- 6-inch double-length elastic bandage
- Tolnaftate© 1% ointment
- 2-inch wide UltraLight© elastic tape, one case
- Second Skin, one jar
- ProWrap underwrap, one case
- Hydrocortisone 1% cream

- 1/8-inch wide Steri-Strips©
- Lidocaine hydrochloride solution, one bottle
- Fluori-Methane, one bottle
- Afrin©, one bottle

MODULE A4—Athletic Training Clinic Equipment—Small (page 18)

- Bioskin Standard Knee Skin (closed patella), size large
- Active ankle brace, right ankle
- Knee immobilizer splint with Velcro closures
- Groin strap—size medium
- Vacuum splints (bag)
- Philadelphia cervical collar
- Crutches—1 pair for an athlete who is 6 feet, 10 inches tall
- Full-length spine board

MODULE B5—Medical Services (page 24)

Community Medical Services

1. Union hospital emergency room
2. Union hospital sports medicine
3. Regional hospital emergency room
4. Regional hospital outpatient room
5. Regional hospital sports medicine/SCORE
6. Dr. Robert Burkle's office
7. VitaCare—Honey Creek Mall

Modules to add

_____

_____

_____

_____

_____

_____

Modules to delete

_____

_____

_____

_____

_____

_____

Appendix C

O/P Examination

O/P examinations have become an integral part of athletic training education at Indiana State University. Completing a comprehensive O/P exam with a score of 85% is an ISU prerequisite for taking the NATA certification exam. NATA requires program directors to verify that certification examination candidates have demonstrated competence in a number of clinical skills before taking the NATA exam. We have chosen to use a comprehensive O/P exam as the means for students to demonstrate their competence in clinical skills. By using this vehicle, students also experience the testing format of the NATA O/P exam and thus are more prepared psychologically for the NATA exam.

Undergraduate students must pass this exam before becoming team trainers. Graduate students must pass it before applying for the NATA certification exam. Both undergraduate and graduate students also may be required to take portions or adaptations of this exam in various athletic training classes, and these adaptations usually will be used as part of the class grade.

The comprehensive O/P exam is administered by both faculty and students. When students administer the exam, a minimum of two, but preferably three, students will administer the exam, each marking the exam sheets independently. Students are welcome to record their exam but must provide the equipment to do so. In the case of a dispute the recording can be used as evidence, but the tape must contain the entire exam and will be reviewed completely. Previous experience has demonstrated that students lose more points than they gain when the tape recording is reviewed.

Cautions

You are cautioned about using this exam exclusively to prepare for the NATA exam. This exam has been, and will continue to be, developed independently from the NATA exam. No effort has been made to determine content of the NATA exam. The formats are somewhat the same, but any similarity in content is strictly coincidental. The intent of the ISU exam is to test you on the content of our educational program. And because our educational program is based on NATA guidelines, there will be some similarity in our exams. We hope that our exam is both broader and more in-depth than the NATA exam; but because we have not seen the NATA exam, and have no interest in doing so, we don't know for sure.

You are also cautioned about using this material exclusively during your preparation for taking an ISU O/P exam. Almost every time this exam has been given during the past 9 years, either new questions have been added or old questions revised. You should prepare by studying the material presented in class. This material is provided to illustrate form and also to neutralize any advantage people think others might have as a result of having old exams from friends.

Grading Exams

Checks are totaled for each question. On some questions the checks are worth a point each, on others a half point each. The net points for each question are added, and the total is divided by the total points possible. The three exams are then averaged. If one of the exams deviates (either higher or lower) from the average of the other two by more than 2.5 times, the deviant score is thrown out and the remaining are averaged.

Instructions to Examiners

1. Ask the examinees if they have any questions. If so, answer them as best as you can. If there is some confusion, write the problem on the cover sheet, and proceed. The problem will be investigated later.

2. The senior examiner (the one who has been there the longest) reads the first question. If the examinee needs clarification, a second examiner should read the question. If further clarification is needed, the third examiner should read the question, then the first again, and so on. Do not explain further, and do not use your own words.

3. If a person does not get a part of the question right, write what they said (or failed to say) on the test booklet.

4. Administer this exam yourself. Don't try to look on other examiners' papers to see if they gave credit on one thing or another. You make the decision. If you need to look up a point in a reference text, do so—in fact, I encourage you to do so; you'll learn more that way. But do not copy another's work. Make your own judgment.

5. Bring reference works and notes to the exam. You won't be able to use them while taking the exam, but you should have them while administering the exam.

6. Don't worry about your decisions. All three examiners will not mark every question exactly the same. But if you are consistent, everything will average out in the end.

7. The person must perform, not tell you what he or she would do. Except in cases where the question indicates otherwise, if the person does not perform during the exam, deduct 5 points from his or her score for that question.

8. Total the number of points for each question immediately after the person finishes it. Write this total on the cover sheet of the test booklet, and add it to the cumulative total. By doing this during the exam, you will not have to take time after the exam is over to total the score.

9. Once the exam is over, pile all three exams together face down and proceed to the next exam. Do not compare scores with the other examiners.

Instructions to the Examinee

These instructions are to be read by examinee before the exam.

1. The supplies intended for your use are on the table. If you believe you need something that is not here, mention how you would use it, and you will be given credit for having done so.

2. Listen to each question carefully. Questions will be repeated as often as you wish, but no further clarifying information will be given.

3. You must act, demonstrate, and perform—not tell what you "would do." Saying "I would . . ." usually will cost you points. During observation, state "I am looking for. . . ."

4. Do not actually use Tufskin, and always use underwrap during this exam. However, indicate whether you would actually use these materials in an actual situation. (This is the one exception to Rule 3.)

5. The subject is not allowed to communicate with you in any way. Often it is imperative that you ask the subject questions, however. Tell what a typical answer would be and act accordingly. During some questions it might be appropriate for you to show what you would do if the subject answered the question in different ways.

6. If you have any questions, ask them before the examination begins.

Sample Questions

Following are sample O/P questions. These can be modified to fit institutional philosophy and teaching emphasis and can be used as templates for developing additional questions.

HEAD AND NECK EVALUATION

Examine an athlete who is down on the field after tackling an opponent. Focus this evaluation primarily on head and neck injuries. (Note to examiners: Give performance points only if the tasks were actually done. Saying "I would . . ." does not count.) You have 7 minutes.

1. CHECK LIFE-THREATENING SITUATIONS
   ___ Breathing
   ___ Heart beating
   ___ Bleeding
   ___ Consciousness
   ___ Cervical spine
   ___ Deal with immediately if present
   ___ TASKS PERFORMED

2. HISTORY OF THE INJURY
   ___ Where hurt
   ___ How hit
   ___ Headache
   ___ Vision
   ___ Nausea
   ___ Tinnitus
   ___ Feeling of dizziness
   ___ Do other body parts hurt?
   ___ TASKS PERFORMED

3. HISTORY OF THE INDIVIDUAL
   ___ Previous head or neck injuries

4. OBSERVATION
   ___ Abnormal position of head and neck
   ___ Lacerations of scalp, head, face
   ___ Fluids from ears, nose, mouth
   ___ TASKS PERFORMED

5. PALPATE
   ___ For pain or point tenderness
   ___ For bumps or deformity
   ___ Scalp and head
   ___ Cervical spine
   ___ Mastoid process
   ___ Extremities
   ___ TASKS PERFORMED

6. TEST STRUCTURAL INTEGRITY
   ___ Pupil reaction (constriction-dilation)
   ___ Pupil tracking
   ___ Check dermatomes both sides
   ___ -Three in hand
   ___ -Two in forearm
   ___ -Two in upper arm
   ___ -Rationale
   ___ TASKS PERFORMED
   ___ Check myotomes both sides
   ___ -Finger apposition, abduction, adduction
   ___ -Finger flexion, extension
   ___ -Wrist flexion, extension
   ___ -Elbow flexion, extension
   ___ -Shoulder abduction and rotation
   ___ -Rationale
   ___ TASKS PERFORMED

7. TEST FUNCTIONAL ACTIVITY
   ___ Memory—obvious things, not date
   ___ Mental confusion—count back by 3, 7
   ___ Neck rotation (while lying on ground)
   ___ Neck flexion, extension (on ground)
   ___ Neck lateral deviation (on ground)
   ___ TASKS PERFORMED

8. DECISION AND ACTION
   ___ Spine board and ambulance if suspect cervical spine injury
   ___ Sit up if OK
   ___ Check balance, pain
   ___ Stand up if OK
   ___ Check balance, pain
   ___ Take off field if OK
   ___ TASKS PERFORMED

9. REEVALUATE
   ___ Arms outstretched
   ___ Finger to nose
   ___ Romberg test
   ___ Heel to knee
   ___ Tandum walk
   ___ TASKS PERFORMED
   ___ Neck motion
   ___ -Active
   ___ -Passive
   ___ -Resistive
   ___ Dermatomes
   ___ Myotomes
   ___ Concussive signs
   ___ TASKS PERFORMED

10. RECORD RESULTS

   ___ ** Give five checks if this is mentioned
   ___ **
   ___ **
   ___ **
   ___ **
   ___

   ___ TOTAL CHECKS

   ___ TOTAL POINTS

(38 possible—each check is worth 1/2 point)

ANKLE EVALUATION

Examine an athlete who complains of a sprained ankle. (Note to examiners: Give performance points only if the tasks were actually done. Saying "I would . . ." does not count.) You have 7 minutes.

1. CHECK LIFE-THREATENING SITUATIONS
   ___ 3 Bs (breathing, beating, bleeding)
   ___ Traumatic shock

2. HISTORY OF THE INJURY
   ___ Rationale
   ___ Where hurt
   ___ When it happened
   ___ How it happened
   ___ Position of foot before injury
   ___ Position of foot after injury
   ___ Questions actually asked

3. HISTORY OF THE INDIVIDUAL
   ___ Rationale
   ___ Previous ankle injuries (when)
   ___ -See physician
   ___ -What rehab
   ___ Questions actually asked

4. OBSERVATION
   ___ Compare opposite sides of body
   ___ Swelling
   ___ Deformity
   ___ TASKS PERFORMED

5. PALPATE
   ___ Tell athlete it will hurt and why
   ___ For pain or point tenderness
   ___ For bumps or deformity
   ___ Start away from suspected injury

   ___ Bones
   ___ Squeeze malleoli
   ___ Rationale
   ___ TASKS PERFORMED
   ___ Deltoid ligaments
   ___ Lateral ligaments
   ___ -All three palpated
   ___ -In correct order
   ___ TASKS PERFORMED

6. TEST STRUCTURAL INTEGRITY
   ___ Sensory nerves
   ___ Motor nerves
   ___ Circulation
   ___ TASKS PERFORMED
   ___ Active ROM
   ___ -Dorsiflexion, plantarflexion
   ___ -Inversion, eversion
   ___ -Rationale
   ___ TASKS PERFORMED
   ___ Passive ROM
   ___ -Eversion
   ___ -Inversion with dorsiflexion
   ___ TASKS PERFORMED
   ___ -Plantarflexion
   ___ -Inversion with plantarflexion
   ___ -Rationale
   ___ TASKS PERFORMED
   ___ Resistive ROM
   ___ -Dorsiflexion
   ___ -Inversion/eversion
   ___ -Plantarflexion
   ___ -Rationale
   ___ TASKS PERFORMED
   ___ Anterior drawer test
   ___ -Hand placement correct
   ___ -Pressure exerted
   ___ -Rationale
   ___ TASKS PERFORMED

7. TEST FUNCTIONAL ACTIVITY
   ___ Only if suspect mild injury
   ___ Walk
   ___ Hop 25 times
   ___ Jog
   ___ Run and cut
   ___ Rationale
   ___ Subject performed tasks

8. DECISION AND ACTION
   ___ If mild injury—tape and play
   ___ If moderate injury—RICES
   ___ If severe—transport to physician

9. REEVALUATE
   ___ After RICEs, if used
   ___ Throughout rehabilitation

10. RECORD RESULTS

   ___ ** Give six checks if mentioned
   ___ ** After the evaluation
   ___ **
   ___ **
   ___ **
   ___ **

   ___ TOTAL CHECKS (72 possible)

   ___ TOTAL POINTS (36 possible)

WRIST EVALUATION

Examine an athlete with wrist pain. (Note to examiners: Give performance points only if the tasks were actually done. Saying "I would . . ." does not count.) You have 7 minutes.

1. CHECK LIFE-THREATENING SITUATIONS

   ___ Traumatic shock

2. HISTORY OF THE INJURY
   ___ Rationale
   ___ Where does it hurt? Point to it.
   ___ When it happened, was it gradual or sudden?
   ___ How did it happen?
   ___ Pain?
   ___ -Sharp
   ___ -Dull
   ___ -Paresthesis
   ___ -Rationale
   ___ Position of hand before/after injury
   ___ -Forced hyperextension, rationale
   ___ -Fall on back of hand, rationale
   ___ Questions actually asked

3. HISTORY OF THE INDIVIDUAL
   ___ Rationale
   ___ Previous wrist injuries (when)
   ___ -See physician
   ___ -What rehab
   ___ Training changes?
   ___ Questions actually asked

4. OBSERVATION
   ___ Compare opposite sides of body
   ___ Swelling
   ___ Deformity
   ___ TASKS PERFORMED

5. PALPATE
   ___ Tell athlete it will hurt and why
   ___ For pain or point tenderness
   ___ Pain move up/down, or in one place?
   ___ Start away from suspected injury
   ___ Radius and ulna
   ___ Carpals (all eight)
   ___ Metacarpals
   ___ Anatomical snuff box
   ___ -Rationale
   ___ Back of wrist
   ___ -Rationale
   ___ TASKS PERFORMED

6. TEST STRUCTURAL INTEGRITY
   ___ Sensory nerves
   ___ Circulation—pinch nail beds
   ___ Allen's test, radial
   ___ Allen's test, ulnar
   ___ TASKS PERFORMED

Active ROM

   ___ -Flexion, extension
   ___ -Radial, ulnar deviation
   ___ -Rationale
   ___ TASKS PERFORMED

Passive ROM

   ___ Flexion, extension
   ___ -Radial, ulnar deviation
   ___ -Rationale
   ___ TASKS PERFORMED

Resistive ROM

   ___ -Flexion, extension
   ___ -Radial, ulnar deviation
   ___ -Rationale
   ___ TASKS PERFORMED
   ___ Finger strength and movement
   ___ Tapping test (over CT)
   ___ -Rationale
   ___ TASKS PERFORMED
   ___ Wrist press
   ___ -Rationale
   ___ TASKS PERFORMED
   ___ Murphy's test
   ___ -Rationale
   ___ TASKS PERFORMED

7. TEST FUNCTIONAL ACTIVITY
___ Only if suspect injury to be mild
___ Use sport-specific activities
___ TASKS PERFORMED

8. DECISION AND ACTION
___ If mild injury, tape and play (no pain)
___ If moderate injury, RICES and immobilize
___ -X-ray
___ If severe, transport to physician

9. REEVALUATE
___ After RICES, if used
___ Throughout rehabilitation

10. RECORD RESULTS
___ ** Give five checks if this is mentioned after the evaluation
___ **
___ **
___ **
___ **
___

___ TOTAL CHECKS/2 = TOTAL POINTS

(38 possible—each check = 1/2 point)

Examiners: Get the next question started!

CRUTCH USE

Prepare an athlete with a sprained ankle to use crutches. For this demonstration, don't worry about removing screws and bolts, but explain how and why you would.

___ With patient lying
___ Adjust length (2-3 inches between axilla and pad)
___ Adjust handpiece (elbow is flexed 20-30 degrees)
___ Confirm adjustment with patient standing

Instruct patient

___ Shoulders do not bear weight—causes crutch palsy
___ Hands bear weight
___ Walking gait assists in maintaining normal gait
___ Crutches take off just enough weight from injured foot
___ Demonstrate gait—actually did it
___ Swing gait—completely remove weight

___ Demonstrate gait—actually did it
___ Demonstrate stairs
___ Upstairs—good leg first
___ Downstairs—crutches first
___ Observe and correct patient—actually did it

___ TOTAL (15)

SLING WITH ELASTIC WRAPS

Using the materials available, apply a sling to the shoulder of an athlete who has a possible glenohumeral dislocation.

___ 6-inch double-length wrap or two single-length wraps
___ Begin around wrist
___ Over opposite shoulder and down back
___ Hand held higher than elbow
___ Hand not held too high (at least 3-4 inches below neck)
___ Wrist firmly supported
___ Elbow held up
___ Humerus held against body
___ Minimal movement
___ Convey feeling of confidence

___ TOTAL (10)

CRYOKINETICS

Demonstrate and explain a cryokinetics program for rehabilitation of a second-degree ankle sprain. Do not use actual ice and water, but tell how you would. Once the subject is performing a specific phase of the procedure, tell what rationale you would use for moving on to the next phase, and then do so. You will receive no points for anything done after 5 minutes from when you start.

___ Evaluate ankle
___ Check response to previous treatment
___ Check contraindications
___ Immerse ankle in ice water
___ Explain pain and adaptation (will not be as painful second time)
___ Encourage patient through pain
___ Ice until numb—20 minutes maximum (must state both)
___ Work non-weight-bearing ROM
___ Work until numbness wears off
___ Ice until renumb—5 minutes maximum
___ Weight-bearing ROM if pain-free

___ Ice until renumb—5 minutes maximum
___ Remove shoe from uninjured foot
___ Stretch heel cord
___ Walk small steps, then large
___ Walk lazy S, then sharp Z
___ Begin strengthening exercises (dorsiflexion and eversion)
___ Jog straight
___ Jog lazy S, then Z
___ Sprint, gradually start and stop
___ Sprint, quickly start and stop
___ Sprint S and Zs
___ Team drills at 50%, 75%, and then full speed
___ Team practice at 50%, 75%, and then full speed
___ Five exercises/bout
___ Progress as fast as possible
___ Pain is guide
___ Advise to apply cold pack if pain returns
___ Put away equipment
___ ** Record results
___ ** 3 points if mentioned
___ **
___ TOTAL (32)

WHIRLPOOL-GENERAL SORENESS

Apply a whirlpool treatment to an athlete who is generally sore after the first week of twice daily practices. Demonstrate all procedures except actually filling the whirlpool and turning it on. Explain, however, when, and how you would fill it and turn it on and off.

PREAPPLICATION

___ Reevaluate injury
___ Review response to previous treatment

___ Explain purpose to patient
___ Check contraindications
___ -
___ -
___ Warn about precautions
___ -
___ -
___ Close the drain
___ Fill whirlpool two-thirds to three-fourths full
___ Temperature 100-108 degrees
___ Check periodically so pool doesn't overfill
___ Check electrical
___ Remove appropriate clothing
___ Turn on turbine before patient gets in

APPLICATION

___ Position patient to about chest-high water
___ Adjust turbine height—must tell how
___ Adjust turbine direction—must tell how
___ Adjust water pressure—must tell how
___ Adjust air flow—must tell how
___ Duration
___ Frequency
___ Turn off turbine before patient gets out

POSTAPPLICATION

___ Arrange next treatment
___ Instruct about activity
___ Clean whirlpool (daily or after every 7-10 treatments)
___ ** Record treatment
___ ** 5 points if mentioned
___ **
___ **
___ **
___ TOTAL (32)

References

Following are the texts that are referred to within the modules. In addition to these references, your institution should have a supplementary list of references and a file of journal reprints or copies for you to refer to (hopefully in or very near your main athletic training clinic). Check with a clinical instructor or faculty athletic trainer.

Allsen PE, Harrison JM, Vance B. 1997. *Fitness for Life*. 6th ed. St. Louis: WCB-McGraw Hill.

American Academy of Orthopaedic Surgeons. 1999. *Athletic Training and Sports Medicine*. 3rd ed. Edited by Robert C. Scheneck Jr. Park Ridge, IL: American Academy of Orthopaedic Surgeons.

American Liver Foundation lay summaries on Hepatitis A, B, and C. Available: **http://www.liverfoundation.org/html/livheal. dir/lhdddox.dir/lhl3dox.fol/lhl3hep.htm**

Anderson MK, Hall SJ, Martin MS. 2000. *Sports Injury Management*. 2nd ed. Philadelphia: Lippincott Williams & Wilkins.

Arnheim DD, Prentice WE. 2000. *Principles of Athletic Training*. 10th ed. New York: McGraw-Hill.

Arnold BL. 1995. A review of selected blood-borne pathogen position statements and federal regulations. *J Athl Train* 30:171-176.

Denegar CR. 2000. *Therapeutic Modalities for Athletic Injuries*. Champaign, IL: Human Kinetics.

Foster DT, Rowedder LJ, Reese SK. 1995. Management of sports-induced skin wounds. *J Athl Train* 30:135-139.

Hillman SK. 2000. *Introduction to Athletic Training*. Champaign, IL: Human Kinetics.

Houglum PA. 2001. *Therapeutic Exercise for Athletic Injuries*. Champaign, IL: Human Kinetics.

Ingersoll CD. 2002. *Research in Athletic Training*. Thorofare, NJ: Slack.

Kisner M, Colby LA. 1996. *Therapeutic Exercise: Foundations and Techniques*. 3rd ed. Philadelphia: Davis.

Knight KL. 1995. *Cryotherapy in Sport Injury Management*. Champaign, IL: Human Kinetics.

Magee DJ. 1997. *Orthopedic Physical Assessment*. 3rd ed. Philadelphia: Saunders.

Martin M, Yates WN Jr. 1998. *Therapeutic Mediations in Sports Medicine*. Baltimore: Williams & Wilkins.

Merten T, Potteiger JA. 1991. Strength training: Proper techniques for the big three. *Athletic Training, Journal of the NATA* 26:295-309.

NATA Position Statements. Available at: **http://www.nata.org/publications/otherpub/ positionstatements.htm**

> Bloodborne Pathogens Guidelines

> Fluid Replacement for Athletes (also in *J Athl Train* 2000; 35:212-224)

> Lightning Safety for Athletics and Recreation. (also in *J Athl Train* 2000; 35:471-477)

Perrin DH. 1993. *Isokinetic Exercise and Assessment*. Champaign, IL: Human Kinetics.

Perrin DH. 1995. *Athletic Taping and Bracing*. Champaign, IL: Human Kinetics.

Pfeiffer RP, Mangus BC. 1998. *Concepts of Athletic Training*. 2nd ed. Boston: Jones and Bartlett.

Prentice WE. 1999a. *Rehabilitation Techniques in Sports Medicine*. 3rd ed. St. Louis: Mosby-Year Book.

Prentice WE. 1999b. *Therapeutic Modalities in Sports Medicine*. 4th ed. St. Louis: Mosby-Year Book.

Rankin JM, Ingersoll CD. 2001. *Athletic Training Management: Concepts and Applications*. New York: McGraw-Hill.

Ray R. 2000. *Management Strategies in Athletic Training*. 2nd ed. Champaign, IL: Human Kinetics.

Rheinecker SB. 1995. Wound management: The occlusive dressing. *J Athl Train* 30:143-146.

Shultz SJ, Houglum PA, Perrin DH. 2000. *Assessment of Athletic Injuries*. Champaign, IL: Human Kinetics.

Starkey C. 1999. *Therapeutic Modalities for Athletic Trainers*. 2nd ed. Philadelphia: Davis.

Starkey C, Ryan JL. 2002. *Evaluation of Orthopedic and Athletic Injuries*. 2nd ed. Philadelphia: Davis.

Tippett SR, Voight ML. 1995. *Functional Progressions for Sport Rehabilitation*. Champaign, IL: Human Kinetics.

Wright KE, Whitehill WR. 1991. *The Comprehensive Manual of Taping and Wrapping Techniques*. Gardner, KS: Cramer.

Other Reference Sources

About the Author

Kenneth L. Knight, PhD, is professor of athletic training at Brigham Young University and a nationally recognized leader in athletic training education. He has been involved in athletic training education for over 32 years as an athletic trainer for high school, junior college, and college teams.

Dr. Knight has taught more than 1,500 students. He was inducted into the NATA Hall of Fame in 2001 and named the NATA Most Distinguished Athletic Trainer in 2000. He received the Sayers "Bud" Miller Outstanding Educator Award in 1995 and the Clancy Medal for Outstanding Research in Athletic Training from the NATA in 1995 and 1997, respectively.

He is also the author of *Cryotherapy: Theory, Technique and Physiology* and *Cryotherapy in Sport Injury Management.*

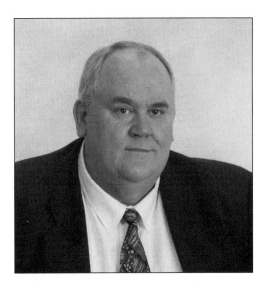